ESSENTIALS OF HAND SURGERY

ESSENTIALS OF HAND SURGERY

Editor

John Gray Seiler III, M.D.

*Clinical Associate Professor
Department of Orthopaedic Surgery
Emory University School of Medicine
Surgeon
Georgia Hand and Microsurgery
Piedmont Hospital
Atlanta, Georgia*

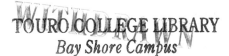
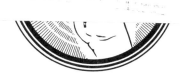

American Society for Surgery of the Hand

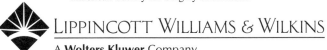

LIPPINCOTT WILLIAMS & WILKINS
A **Wolters Kluwer** Company

Philadelphia · Baltimore · New York · London
Buenos Aires · Hong Kong · Sydney · Tokyo

BS

Acquisitions Editor: Robert Hurley
Developmental Editor: Tanya Lazar
Production Editor: Tom Wang
Manufacturing Manager: Tim Reynolds
Cover Designer: Wanda Kossack
Compositor: Lippincott Williams & Wilkins Desktop Division
Printer: Edwards Brothers

Printed in the USA

Library of Congress Cataloging-in-Publication Data
Essentials of hand surgery / edited by John Gray Seiler III.—1st ed.
    p.;   cm.
Includes index.
ISBN 0-7817-3585-8
1. Hand—Surgery.   2. Hand—Wounds and injuries.   I. Seiler, John Gray.   II. Amer-
ican Society for Surgery of the Hand.
[DNLM: 1. Hand—Surgery.   2. hand—anatomy & histology.   3. Hand Injuries—
diagnosis. WE 830 E78 2001]
RD559.E78 2001
617.575059—dc21   2001041364

10 9 8 7 6 5 4 3 2 1

10/29/23

To my wife, June, and our children, John Gray, Stuart, Virginia, and William.
For their love, support, and patience.

Contents

Contributing Authors

Mark E. Baratz, M.D. *Professor, Department of Orthopaedic Surgery, MCP —Hahnemann University, Philadelphia, Pennsylvania; and Vice Chairman, Department of Orthopaedic Surgery, Director, Division of Hand and Upper Extremity Surgery, Allegheny General Hospital, Pittsburgh, Pennsylvania*

Michael S. Bednar, M.D. *Associate Professor, Department of Orthopaedic Surgery and Rehabilitation, Loyola University at Chicago, Maywood, Illinois*

Leon S. Benson, M.D. *Assistant Professor of Clinical Orthopaedic Surgery, Department of Orthopaedic Surgery, Northwestern University, Chicago, Illinois; and Attending Orthopaedic Surgeon, Hand and Upper Extremity Surgery, Illinois Bone and Joint Institute, Glenview, Illinois*

Scott H. Kozin, M.D. *Associate Professor, Department of Orthopaedic Surgery, Temple University; and Hand Surgeon, Shriners Hospital for Children, Philadelphia, Pennsylvania*

Donald H. Lee, M.D. *Associate Professor, Division of Orthopaedic Surgery, University of Alabama at Birmingham, Birmingham, Alabama*

Mark S. Lemel, M.D. *Clinical Assistant Professor, Department of Orthopaedics, University of Florida Health Science Center Jacksonville, and Orthopaedic Hand Surgeon, North Florida Hand Surgeons, St. Vincent's Medical Center, Jacksonville, Florida*

Peter M. Murray, M.D. *Associate Professor, Department of Orthopaedic Surgery, Division of Hand and Microvascular Surgery, Mayo Graduate School of Medicine, Rochester, Minnesota; and Senior Associate Consultant, The Mayo Clinic, Jacksonville, Florida*

Matthew D. Putnam, M.D. *Physician, Department of Orthopaedic Surgery, University of Minnesota, Minneapolis, Minnesota*

Mitchell B. Rotman, M.D. *Associate Professor, Director of Hand Surgery, Department of Orthopaedic Surgery, St. Louis University, St. Louis, Missouri*

Craig S. Williams, M.D. *Clinical Assistant Professor, Department of Orthopaedic Surgery, Northwestern University, Chicago, Illinois; and Attending Orthopaedic Surgeon, Hand and Upper Extremity Surgery, Illinois Bone and Joint Institute, Des Plaines, Illinois*

Preface

Essentials in Hand Surgery is a multi-authored textbook that has been developed by an *ad hoc* committee of the American Society for Surgery of the Hand. This book has been created to provide immediate access to basic information about the diagnosis and initial treatment of hand surgery problems. The information contained within the text has been distilled from the practices of knowledgeable and experienced hand surgeons.

A significant amount of the text is devoted to hand anatomy and physical examination of the hand because anatomy is so important to the discipline of hand surgery. Readers who are new to the specialty will find these chapters invaluable for evaluation of patients with hand problems. The remainder of the text is devoted to the evaluation and treatment of common conditions.

We hope you will find this textbook useful for you and the treatment of your patients.

John Gray Seiler III, M.D.

1

Embryology

The clinician involved in the care of children with congenital anomalies must possess a basic understanding of embryogenesis, limb formation, and inheritance patterns. The sequencing of the human genome and investigation into the molecular basis of limb development have provided new information regarding the causes of limb malformation. Advances in genomic and proteomic research have outlined the relationship between underlying gene(s) abnormalities and limb malformation. Genetic evaluation is quickly becoming part of the standard evaluation. In the future, genetic manipulation may prevent certain limb deformities and offer hope to families afflicted with genetic idiosyncrasies.

Embryogenesis of the upper extremity refers to formation of the limb 4 to 8 weeks after fertilization. The majority of upper extremity congenital anomalies occur during this 4-week period of rapid limb development. Limb bud development is initiated by outgrowth of the underlying mesoderm along the axis of the embryo into the overlying ectoderm. A thickened layer of ectoderm (apical ectodermal ridge) condenses over the limb bud and acts as a signaling center to guide the underlying mesoderm to differentiate into appropriate structures. The limb develops in a proximal to distal direction and the apical ectodermal ridge (AER) is responsible for this process. Loss of the AER during embryogenesis results in limb truncation and congenital amputation (Fig. 1). The AER also secretes proteins that influence the development of the underlying tissues. As the hand develops, the AER fragments around the hand paddle, which results in longitudinal interdigital necrosis between the digits. Failure of the AER to separate is the most prevalent explanation for syndactyly.

A second signaling center, the zone of polarizing activity (ZPA), which is responsible for anterior to posterior (radioulnar) development resides within the posterior margin of the limb bud. The hedgehog pathway is located within the ZPA and the signaling molecule necessary for limb orientation is the Sonic hedgehog compound. Duplication of the ZPA into the anterior portion of the limb bud of chick embryos yields digital replication of the ulnar digits along the radial side of the hand, similar to a mirror hand anomaly (Fig. 2). A third signaling center, the Wnt pathway (Wingless type) resides in the dorsal ectoderm

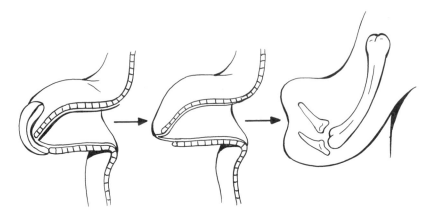

FIG. 1. Removal of the apical ectodermal ridge during limb development results in limb truncation.

and secretes factors that induce the underlying mesoderm to adopt dorsal characteristics. This process mediates the development of dorsal to ventral axis configuration. Mice lacking this pathway have duplicated palms. The AER, ZPA, and Wnt pathway all function in a coordinated effort to ensure proper limb patterning and growth during embryogenesis. Abnormalities of these crucial areas directly affect limb formation and indirectly prohibit adequate functioning of the remaining signaling centers.

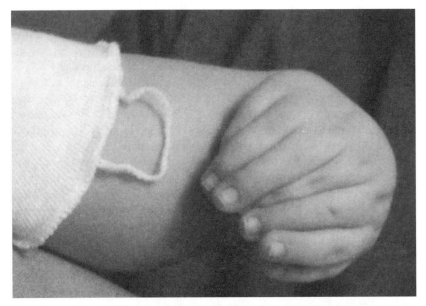

FIG. 2. Mirror hand anomaly with duplication of the ulnar digits along the radial side of the hand.

The arm and forearm appear before the hand plate, which appears by 5-weeks gestation in the form of a paddle covered by the AER. Condensation of the mesoderm forms the skeletal anlage, which eventually undergoes initial chondrification and subsequent ossification. Nerves and vessels permeate into the developing extremity during the fifth through eighth weeks of gestation. Joint formation begins with the condensation of chondrocyte precursors along dense plates as a precursor to joint articulation. Subsequent joint cavitation ensues with formation of a joint cavity that requires motion for continued joint formation. Embryogenesis is complete and all limb structures are present by the eighth week. Subsequently, the fetal period commences with differential growth of existing structures; this process continues until birth.

SELECTED REFERENCES

Bamshad M, Watkins WS, Dixon ME, et al. Reconstructing the history of human limb development: lessons from birth defects. Pediatr Res 1999;45:291—299.
Beatty E. Upper limb tissue differentiation in the human embryo. Hand Clin 1985;1:391–403.
Daluiski A, Yi SE, Lyons KM. The molecular control of upper extremity development: implications for congenital hand anomalies. J Hand Surg 2001;26A:8–22.
Riddle RD, Tabin CJ. How limbs develop. Sci Am 1999;280:74–79.

2

Anatomy

TERMINOLOGY

The hand and digits are described using standard terminology (Fig. 1). They are composed of a dorsal surface, a volar or palmar surface, and radial and ulnar borders. The palm is divided into thenar, midpalm, and hypothenar areas. The thenar area contains the small muscles of the thumb and is called the thenar eminence. The hypothenar area contains the small muscles of the small finger and is called the hypothenar eminence. The digits are designated as the thumb, index, middle or long, ring, and small digits. Each finger has a proximal, middle, and distal phalanx. Each finger also has three joints: the metacarpophalangeal (MCP), the proximal interphalangeal (PIP), and the distal interphalangeal (DIP) joints. The thumb has only two phalanges (proximal and distal) and two joints (MCP and interphalangeal joints). The MCP, PIP, and DIP joints are protected from injury by stabilizing structures. Collateral ligaments protect both sides and a volar plate stabilizes the undersurface of each joint.

Hand motion also is described according to standard terminology (Fig. 2). The thumb is positioned perpendicularly to the fingers, and flexion/extension is in this plane. Abduction of the thumb can either be out of the palm (palmar abduction) or in the plane of the hand (planar or radial abduction). Thumb opposition is a combination of thumb rotation (pronation), palmar abduction, and flexion. A sagittal line through the third ray defines the center of the hand. Finger abduction/adduction is described using this reference coordinate; therefore, abduction is away from the long finger and adduction is toward it. The long finger itself is able to abduct away from this line in a radial or ulnar direction.

INTEGUMENT/FASCIA

The palmar and dorsal skins are distinctively different with respect to structure and function. The palmar skin is thick with fibrous septa connecting the

4

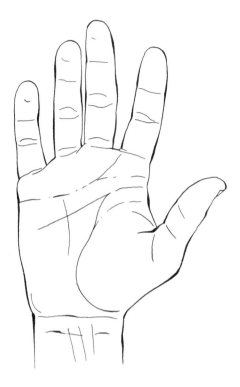

A

FIG. 1. A and B: Surface anatomy of the hand.

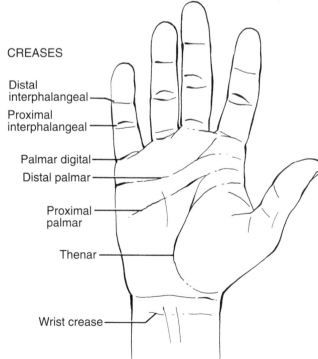

CREASES

Distal
interphalangeal

Proximal
interphalangeal

Palmar digital

Distal palmar

Proximal
palmar

Thenar

Wrist crease

B

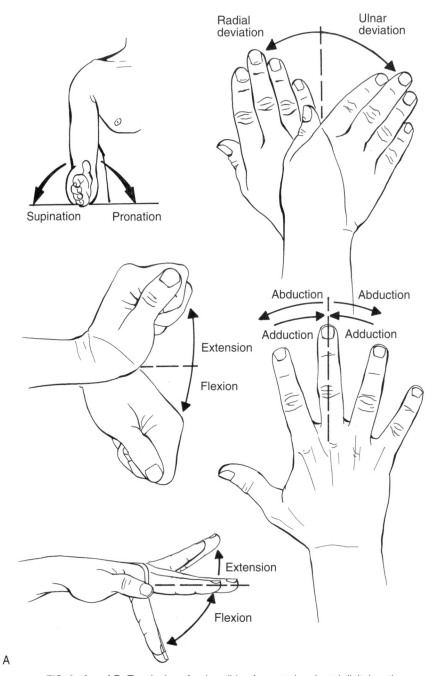

FIG. 2. A and B: Terminology for describing forearm, hand, and digital motion.

Radial deviation

Ulnar deviation

Supination   Pronation

Extension

Flexion

Abduction   Abduction

Adduction   Adduction

Extension

Flexion

A

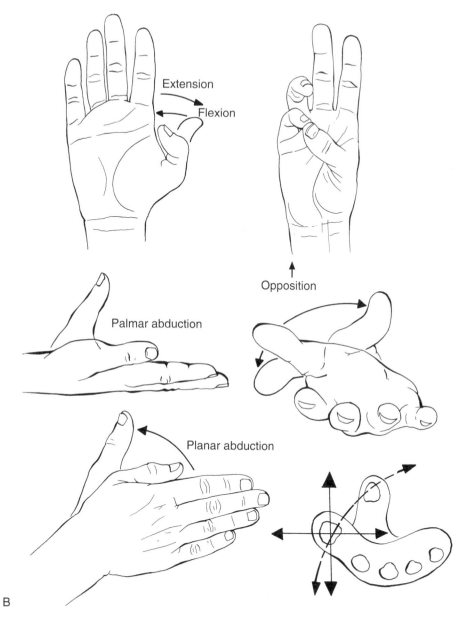

FIG. 2. *Continued.*

skin to the underlying fascia. This attachment limits motion and provides a stable platform for grasping and manipulation of objects. In contrast, the dorsal skin is loose with areolar tissue between the skin and extensor tendons. This laxity creates the dorsal subcutaneous space for lymphatic and venous drainage. This structural difference accounts for the dorsal hand swelling seen during infection even when the source is located on the palmar side of the hand.

The palmar fascia of the hand provides a stable platform for the skin and protects the underlying structures (Fig. 3). This fascia is also the insertion site for the palmaris longus tendon, allowing this muscle to flex the wrist. A septum extending from the palmar aponeurosis to the third metacarpal divides the recesses of the hand into spaces (Fig. 4). These spaces are deeper and different from the palmar surface areas described earlier. The thenar space is located to the radial side of the septum and the midpalmar space is situated on the ulnar side. These spaces can be infected primarily or secondarily following flexor tenosynovitis of the digits.

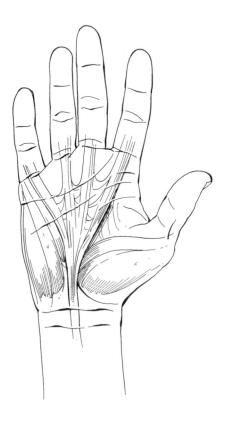

FIG. 3. Palmar fascia of the hand provides stability and protection to the hand.

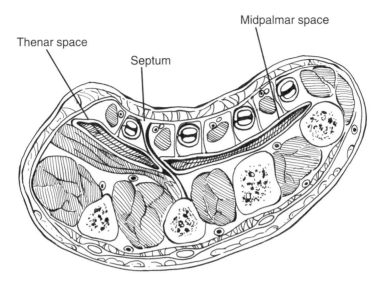

FIG. 4. Transverse section demonstrating septum from palmar fascia to third metacarpal, which divides hand into thenar and midpalmar spaces.

BLOOD SUPPLY

The radial and ulnar arteries supply the hand and digits by a series of arches (Fig. 5). The radial artery is located between the brachioradialis and flexor carpi radialis tendons at the wrist. The artery splits into two branches, with the larger dorsal branch coursing under the first dorsal compartment, through the anatomic snuffbox, between the index and thumb metacarpals, and into the recesses of the palm to form the greater part of the deep palmar arch. A smaller palmar branch travels over the flexor carpi radialis tendon, beneath or through the thenar muscles, and forms the radial component of the superficial palmar arch. The ulnar artery is located lateral to the ulnar nerve at the wrist and adjacent to the flexor carpi ulnaris tendon. The nerve and artery course into Guyon's canal, which is bordered by the pisiform and hook of the hamate. The floor of Guyon's canal is the transverse carpal ligament (TCL) and the roof is the volar carpal ligament (Fig. 6). The artery splits into two branches with the larger branch forming the main constituent of the superficial palmar arch. A smaller branch passes deep to connect with the radial artery and form the deep palmar arch.

A line drawn across the palm parallel to the fully abducted thumb (Kaplan's cardinal line) approximates the location of the superficial palmar arch. This arch is located just past the distal edge of the TCL. The deep palmar arch is located one centimeter proximal to the superficial palmar arch and is beneath the flexor tendons. Although considerable variability exists, the superficial palmar arch typically provides palmar blood vessels to the index (ulnar side), long, ring, and small fingers, whereas the deep palmar arch supplies blood ves-

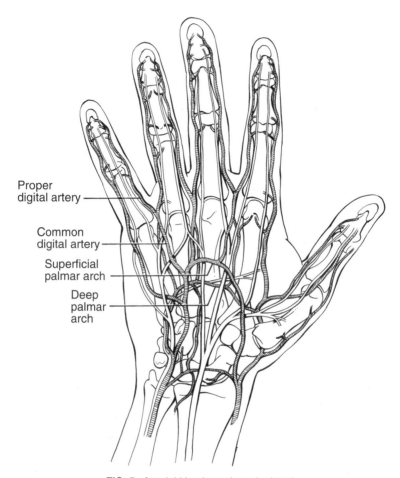

Proper
digital artery

Common
digital artery

Superficial
palmar arch

Deep
palmar
arch

FIG. 5. Arterial blood supply to the hand.

sels to the thumb and index digit (radial side) (Fig. 5). Common digital arteries originate from the superficial palmar arch and travel within the index-long,
long-ring, and ring-small interspaces. These vessels divide into proper digital
arteries that continue along the sides of the digits. The proper digital artery to
the ulnar side of the small finger originates directly from the superficial arch.
The proper digital artery to the radial side of the index finger originates from
the deep palmar arch. The vascular supply to the thumb is from digital
branches that originate as a common trunk (princeps pollicis artery) from the
deep palmar arch. The deep arch also provides metacarpal branches that join
the common digital arteries just proximal to their bifurcation into proper components.

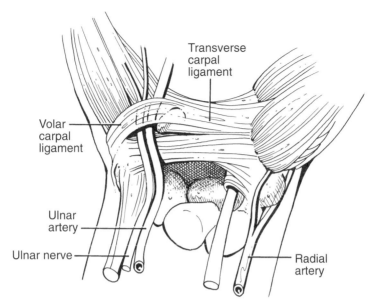

FIG. 6. The transverse carpal ligaments forms the roof to the carpal tunnel and the floor to Guyon's canal.

NERVES

The radial, median, and ulnar nerves supply the sensibility and motor innervation to the hand and forearm. The radial nerve enters the forearm between the two heads of the supinator muscle. The radial nerve innervates the brachioradialis and extensor carpi radialis longus, prior to dividing into the posterior interosseous and radial sensory nerves.

The posterior interosseous nerve innervates the wrist, finger, and thumb extensor muscles, whereas the radial sensory nerve travels down the forearm beneath the brachioradialis muscle adjacent to the radial artery. Subsequently, the sensory nerve passes dorsally beneath the brachioradialis at its musculotendinous junction to provide sensibility to the dorsoradial aspect of the hand and dorsum of the thumb, index, and long digits. The lateral antebrachial cutaneous nerve, which is the terminal branch of the musculocutaneous nerve, also supplies sensibility to this aspect of the hand; therefore, altered sensibility in this area can be from injury to the radial sensory and/or lateral antebrachial cutaneous nerves.

The median nerve enters the forearm between the two heads of the pronator teres muscle. The median nerve travels down the forearm between the flexor digitorum superficialis and profundus muscles to enter the carpal tunnel. Along its course, the anterior interosseous nerve branches from the median nerve to provide innervation to the flexor pollicis longus, flexor digitorum profundus to the index, and the pronator quadratus muscles. The median nerve proper provides innervation to the flexor carpi radialis, pronator teres, flexor digitorum superficialis, palmaris longus (absent in 10% to 15% of individuals), and flexor digitorum profundus to the long finger. The palmar cutaneous branch arises from the median nerve 5 cm proximal to the wrist joint and supplies sensibility to the thenar eminence. Just proximal to the wrist, the median nerve becomes superficial and travels within the carpal tunnel. A recurrent motor branch originates from the central or radial portion of the median nerve during its passage through the carpal tunnel (Fig. 5). The recurrent branch usually passes distal to the TCL to innervate the thenar muscles. Uncommonly, the nerve can also pass through the TCL (5% to 7% of individuals). The median nerve terminates into multiple sensory branches, which supply sensibility to the thumb, index, long, and ring (radial side) fingers. The sensory branches to the radial side of the index and radial side of the long possess a minor motor component and send a small branch that innervates the adjacent lumbrical muscle.

The ulnar nerve enters the forearm between the two heads of the flexor carpi ulnaris muscle. In the forearm, the ulnar nerve innervates the flexor carpi ulnaris and flexor digitorum profundus to the ring and small fingers. A large dorsal ulnar sensory nerve exits the ulnar nerve proximal to the wrist and courses dorsally at the level of the ulnar styloid. This sensory nerve provides sensibility to the ulnar portion of the hand and dorsum of the small and ring (ulnar side) fingers. The ulnar nerve proper, residing medial to the ulnar artery, enters Guyon's canal and provides a motor branch to the hypothenar muscles. A deep motor branch passes around the hook of the hamate to innervate the interossei, ulnar lumbricals, flexor pollicis brevis (deep head), and the adductor pollicis muscles. The ulnar nerve terminates into sensory branches that supply the small and ring (ulnar side) fingers.

MUSCLE/TENDON

The muscles and tendons about the hand originate in the forearm (extrinsic) or within the hand itself (intrinsic). The extrinsic extensor muscles generate tendons that align within compartments along the dorsum of the wrist (Fig. 7). The extensor retinaculum is a 2-cm band that extends from the radial to the ulnar side of the wrist. This retinaculum is a strong pulley that holds the tendons close to the underlying bone. The relationship allows the tendons to fully extend the digits with an efficient amount of tendon excursion. The retinaculum sends septa to the underlying bone, which form six distinct compartments. The first compartment contains the abductor pollicis longus and extensor pollicis brevis tendons that attach to the base of the thumb metacarpal and base of the proximal phalanx, respectively. The second compartment holds the extensor carpi radialis longus and brevis, which insert onto the base of the second and third metacarpal. Within the third compartment, the extensor pollicis longus travels obliquely (45

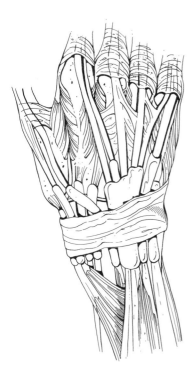

FIG. 7. Extensor tendon compartments along the dorsum of the wrist.

degrees) around Lister's tubercle to form part of the thumb extensor hood and attach to the base of the distal phalanx. The fourth compartment contains the extensor digitorum communis and extensor indicis proprius tendons that form part of the extensor apparatus to the digits and primarily insert into the base of the middle phalanx (central slip). On the dorsum of the hand, the extensor digitorum communis tendons are connected by juncture tendinae. The fifth compartment overlies the distal radioulnar joint and houses the extensor digit minimi, which provides independent extension to the small finger and attaches into the extensor apparatus. The extensor indicis proprius and extensor digit minimi are located ulnar to their extensor communis counterpart. The sixth compartment secures the extensor carpi ulnaris in position about the ulna during its route to the base of the fifth metacarpal.

The carpal tunnel forms the primary compartment along the palmar aspect of the wrist (Fig. 8). The carpal bones form the walls of the carpal tunnel and the overlying TCL constitutes the roof. The TCL attaches to the scaphoid tubercle and trapezial ridge on the radial side and the hook of the hamate and pisiform on the ulnar side. The TCL also forms the floor of Guyon's canal, which contains the ulnar artery and nerve. Nine tendons and the median nerve are within the carpal tunnel. The flexor digitorum superficialis tendons lie just ulnar to the

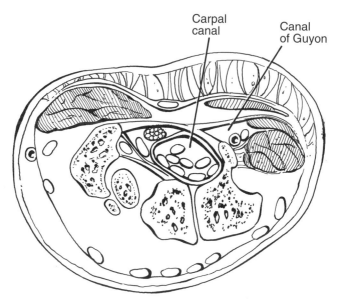

FIG. 8. Transverse section of the carpal tunnel.

nerve and are separated into two layers. The long and ring superficialis tendons lie more palmar than the index and small. The flexor digitorum profundus tendons, which are arranged in a single plane, are beneath the flexor digitorum superficialis. The flexor digitorum superficialis tendons attach to the base of the middle phalanx, and the flexor digitorum profundus tendons insert into the base of the distal phalanx. Along their course, the flexor digitorum superficialis tendons divide into two parts (Camper's chiasm) to permit passage of the flexor digitorum profundus tendons. The flexor pollicis longus runs deep to the median nerve along the radial border of the carpal tunnel and attaches to the distal phalanx of the thumb.

The primary wrist flexors do not reside within the carpal tunnel. The flexor carpi radialis travels in an adjacent separate fibroosseous tunnel en route to insertion at the base of the index and long metacarpals. The flexor carpi ulnaris travels palmar to the carpal tunnel and attaches to the base of the small metacarpal. The flexor carpi ulnaris tendon encompasses the pisiform (a sesamoid bone), which forms the medial wall of Guyon's canal.

The hand muscles are divided into three general groups: the thenar eminence, hypothenar eminence, and hand itself. The thenar muscles are the opponens pollicis, flexor pollicis brevis, and abductor pollicis brevis, and the recurrent branch of the median nerve innervates all. The flexor pollicis brevis muscle receives dual innervation from both the recurrent branch (superficial head) and the deep motor branch of the ulnar nerve (deep head). The hypothenar muscles are the opponens digiti quinti, flexor digiti quinti, and abductor digiti quinti; the ulnar nerve innervates all. All thenar and hypothenar muscles except the abductor digiti quinti originate in part from the transverse carpal ligament. In addition, all have insertions distal to the MCP joint and may contribute to the extensor apparatus, except the opponens muscles. The opponens pollicis and opponens digiti quinti insert along the borders of the metacarpals to rotate the hands for opposition. The thenar and hypothenar muscles function as prime movers of the thumb and small finger and their coordinated activity allows fine manipulation of objects and force production during grasp and pinch.

The muscles within the hand are the interossei, lumbricals, and adductor pollicis. The deep branch of the ulnar nerve innervates all these muscles. There are four bipennate dorsal interossei that originate from adjacent sides of the metacarpals and have similar structure (Fig. 9). For example, the first interosseus muscle originates from the thumb and index metacarpals and inserts into two points. One site of attachment is into the radial side of the index proximal phalanx, which provides abduction away from the third ray. The second insertion site is into the extensor apparatus, which provides MCP joint flexion and interphalangeal joint extension. The second dorsal interosseous muscle originates from the adjacent sides of the index and long fingers, the third from the long and ring fingers, and the fourth from the ring and small fingers. The dorsal interossei provide abduction of the finger along with MCP joint flexion and interphalangeal joint extension. There are three smaller unipennate palmar interossei that originate from a single metacarpal. The first arises from the ulnar side of the index metacarpal and inserts with dual insertion sites similar to the dorsal interossei

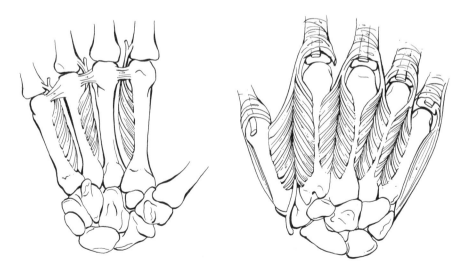

FIG. 9. The four bipennate dorsal interossei and the three unipennate palmar interossei.

(i.e., proximal phalanx and extensor apparatus). These attachment sites provide adduction toward the long finger along with MCP joint flexion and interphalangeal joint extension. The second and third interossei function in the same way and originate from the radial side of the ring and small metacarpals, respectively. Each interossei can be encircled in a discrete fascial compartment. The four lumbrical muscles originate within the hand from the radial side of the flexor digitorum profundus tendons. These muscles course beneath the intermetacarpal ligament and contribute to the lateral bands.

The adductor pollicis muscle is similar to a palmar interosseus in terms of function. The adductor pollicis originates from the third metacarpal and inserts into multiple sites, including the base of the proximal phalanx and extensor apparatus (forming the adductor aponeurosis). Contraction of the adductor pollicis muscle produces an intrinsic response with MCP joint flexion, interphalangeal joint extension, and thumb adduction.

The flexor tendons of the digits enter a fibroosseous tunnel at the level of the MCP joint, which is referred to as the flexor sheath (Fig. 10). The sheath is thickened at various strategic points to produce strong annular pulleys that position the tendons close to the underlying bone. This arrangement makes the best use of tendon excursion and allows full flexion and extension. Loss of the A2 or A4 pulley allows the flexor tendons to bow away from the bone, which increases the flexion moment arm, causes a digital flexion contracture, and prohibits full flexion at the digit. The second annular (A2) pulley overlies the proximal phalanx and the fourth annular (A4) is positioned over the middle phalanx. Cruciate pulleys are interdigitated between the annular pulleys and are less critical for function. These pulleys have two crossing bands and are more flexible than the annular configuration. During digital flexion and extension, the cruciate pulleys compress and stretch (like an accordion), which allows allow full motion. The

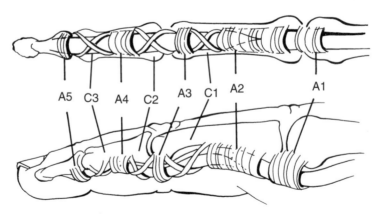

FIG. 10. The annular and cruciate pulleys of the flexor tendon sheath.

flexor tendon sheath is lined by modified fibroblasts, which lubricate the tendon to minimize friction and contributes to tendon nutrition.

The extensor apparatus over the dorsum of the fingers deserves special mention (Fig. 11). The extensor digitorum communis tendons pass over the MCP joint and are held in position by the sagittal hood, which wraps around the MCP joint to attach to the volar plate. The extensor digitorum communis extends the MCP joint by pulling on the sagittal fibers of the hood that are attached to the palmar plate, which lifts the proximal phalanx. Distal to the MCP joint, the extensor digitorum communis divides into three parts. The central portion continues distally and attaches to the base of the middle phalanx (central slip). The marginal slips of the extensor digitorum communis tendon contribute to the lat-

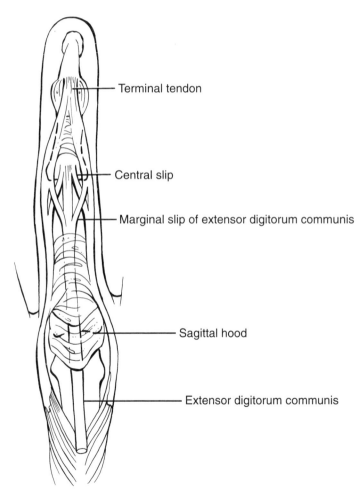

Terminal tendon

Central slip

Marginal slip of extensor digitorum communis

Sagittal hood

Extensor digitorum communis

FIG. 11. Extensor apparatus over the dorsum of the digits.

eral bands, which are formed primarily by the tendons of the interossei and lumbricals. The lateral bands terminate at the base of the distal phalanx and are responsible for PIP and DIP joint extension.

OSSEOUS/LIGAMENTS

The carpus or wrist consists of eight bones organized into two rows (Fig. 12). The proximal row includes the scaphoid, lunate, and triquetrum. The distal row consists of the trapezium, trapezoid, capitate, and hamate. The pisiform is actually a sesamoid bone within the flexor carpi ulnaris and does not participate in carpal motion. The bones within each row are held together by interosseus ligaments, which provide linkage and allow a variable amount of motion. The integrity of these ligaments is critical to normal wrist motion (carpal kinematics), especially because no tendons attach directly to the carpal bones. Wrist flexion/extension is a combination of radiocarpal motion and movement between the carpal rows (midcarpal joint). Radial and ulnar deviation requires coordination between the proximal and distal rows as they move in opposite directions during this movement. Disruption of the integrity of the interosseous

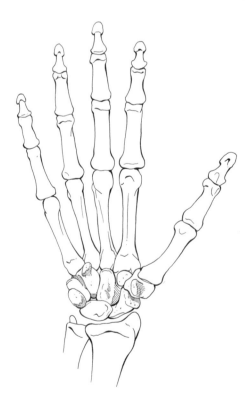

FIG. 12. Bony anatomy of the wrist and hand.

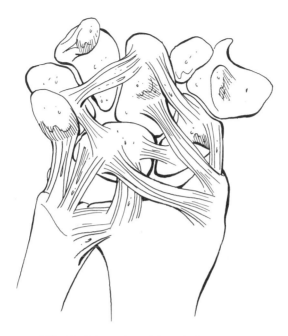

FIG. 13. Palmar view of the wrist ligaments.

ligaments often leads to loss of synchrony between adjacent carpal bones, altered wrist motion, and pain.

The wrist also possesses ligaments that connect the radius to the carpus and are called extrinsic ligaments. The palmar extrinsic ligaments are more important to wrist stability and motion than are the dorsal ligaments (Fig. 13). The triangular fibrocartilage complex (TFCC) originates from the radius and attaches to the base of the ulnar styloid. The dorsal and volar radioulnar ligaments are thickenings of the TFCC and provide stability to the distal radioulnar joint.

NAILBED

The nail plate originates 5 to 7 mm proximal to the nail fold in the germinal nail matrix (Fig. 14). This is responsible for nail length. The visible nail bed, or sterile matrix, thickens the nail and provides an adherent surface that stabilizes the nail. The dorsal nail fold, or eponychium, adds the smooth shiny surface of the nail. The fingertip skin or hyponychium is very sensate. Fibrous septae deep to the skin surface provide traction for gripping and stabilize the skin at the tip of the digit. Deep to the nail bed a broad-based bony tuft of the distal phalanx provides skeletal support for pinch and grasp. The flexor and extensor tendons insert proximally on the distal phalanx away from the nail area.

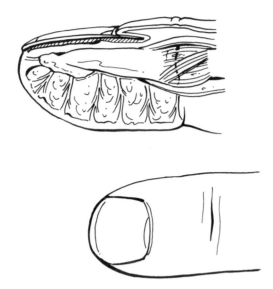

FIG. 14. Nail bed and tip.

SUGGESTED READINGS

Bishop AT, Gabel G, Carmichael SW. Flexor carpi radialis tendinitis. Part I: operative anatomy. J Bone Joint Surg Am 1994;76:1009–1014.

Hoppenfeld S, deBoer P. Surgical exposures in orthopaedics. The anatomic approach. JB Lippincott, Philadelphia, 1984, pp. 141–208.

Kozin SH. Anatomy of the recurrent motor branch of the median nerve. J Hand Surg 1998;23A:852–858.

Kozin SH, Clark P, Porter S, Thoder JJ. The contribution of the intrinsic muscles to grip and pinch strength. J Hand Surg 1999;24A:64–72.

Lampe EW. Clinical symposia. Surgical anatomy of the hand. Ciba-Geigy Corporation, Summit, New Jersey, 1998;40:3–36.

Rotman MB, Manske PR. Anatomic relationships of an endoscopic carpal tunnel device to surrounding structures. J Hand Surg [Am] 1993;18:442–450.

Smith RJ. Balance and kinetics of the fingers under normal and pathological conditions. Clin Orthop 1974;104:92–111.

3

History

The patient's history can be the most important tool in developing an accurate diagnosis. The prudent physician is both thorough and organized. The history should not only detail the patient's current complaint, but also document other elements of the patient's medical history, which can be of great significance for interpreting the current problem and choosing treatment options.

The history can be separated into several categories:

1. Patient demographics
2. Current complaint
3. Medical history
4. Allergies and medications
5. Social history

The time and date of the interview should be clearly documented as the history is taken.

PATIENT DEMOGRAPHICS

Basic information that should be recorded includes the patient's name, age, sex, occupation, and hand dominance.

CURRENT COMPLAINT

As much detail as possible should be obtained about the patient's current problem. First, identify the presenting symptoms. It can be helpful to ask about the following complaints:

Pain
Numbness
Tingling (paresthesias)
Weakness
Discoloration
Coldness

Clumsiness or poor coordination
Clicking or snapping

These symptoms should be characterized further by the following descriptors: *location, intensity, duration, frequency, radiation,* and *associated symptoms.* A thorough history also documents what activities or treatments make the current complaint better or worse.

It is important to record the mechanism, time, and place where an injury occurred (i.e., home or workplace). Mechanism of injury should include as many details as possible, because such details may determine outcome. For example, a crushing- or exploding-type injury that produces amputation of the hand has a much poorer prognosis than an amputation caused by a sharp power saw. It can be helpful to know the position of the hand or extremity at the exact moment of injury and whether any treatment has been administered. The physician should also determine whether the patient has had any previous injuries that have had an effect on the current injury. The time of their last meal and tetanus immunization should also be noted for trauma patients.

MEDICAL HISTORY

The patient's general health can influence both diagnosis and treatment. It is important to know about the presence of diabetes; cardiac, pulmonary, or renal disease; and any history of rheumatologic or dermatologic problems. All patients requiring surgery should be specifically questioned about both personal *and* family history of problems with bleeding and anesthesia. The patient's prior surgical history should be recorded.

ALLERGIES AND MEDICATIONS

This part of the history documents which medications the patient is taking and which medication or food allergies are present. Many patients who are allergic to shellfish also react to intravenous iodine-contrast media.

SOCIAL HISTORY

Social history includes the patient's tobacco and alcohol use. It is also important to note any history of substance abuse, hepatitis infection, or HIV infection. The patient's hobbies and sports interests are also included in the social history because these activities frequently influence treatment decisions.

4

Physical Examination
of the Hand

Accurate diagnosis of hand problems relies on a careful physical examination. The examiner's skills improve with practice, especially if the examination is organized into a routine that is thorough and efficient. It is wise to follow a specific protocol when examining patients. All clinicians develop their own style when interacting with patients. The best formats are simple, systematic, thorough, and comprehensive.

The physical examination of the hand is organized into eight elements:

    I. Inspection
   II. Palpation
  III. Range of motion assessment
       A. Active motion
       B. Passive motion
  IV. Stability assessment
   V. Muscle and tendon assessment
       A. Flexor
          1. Intrinsic
          2. Extrinsic
       B. Extensor
          1. Intrinsic
          2. Extrinsic
       C. Intrinsic
       D. Extrinsic
  VI. Nerve assessment
 VII. Vascular assessment
VIII. Integument assessment

Although it is possible to consider the elements separately, the examiner must understand the interrelationships among these systems to reach accurate conclusions.

Ideally, the patient should be seated, facing directly opposite the examiner. It is helpful to use a narrow table between patient and doctor. This not only allows the patient to comfortably rest the forearm, but also serves as a flat surface that can facilitate some elements of the physical examination.

INSPECTION

While inspecting the hand, the examiner should look specifically for:

Discoloration
Deformity
Muscular atrophy
Trophic changes (sweat pattern, hair growth)
Swelling
Wounds or scars

Inspecting both of the patient's hands at the same time is helpful, especially if the problem is unilateral, because the normal hand makes a good reference for comparison.

Discoloration may indicate a wide variety of problems. Skin infections (cellulitis) commonly present with patches of redness with proximal streaking. Vascular inflow problems (arterial blockage) produce white discoloration distally, whereas outflow problems (venous blockage) commonly result in blue or purple, swollen fingers. Hematomas from recent trauma produce patches of purple or blue that eventually change to green and then yellow before they disappear. Some skin cancers produce a dark spot in the skin or a black line in the nailbed. Other skin diseases that have typical appearances are fungal infections, psoriasis, and viral infections.

Inspection for *deformity* involves looking for asymmetry, unusual angulation, and rotation. Broken bones are often noticeable as a crooked finger. The digital alignment should be checked in full flexion and full extension. The fingers should fold up into the hand when the patient makes a fist, with the fingertips all gently converging toward a common point on the wrist. Malrotated phalangeal or metacarpal fractures are obvious when the patient flexes the fingers, because the affected digit will cross over (or under) an adjacent digit. Comparison with the opposite hand can be helpful. Sometimes after comparing both hands, it becomes clear that what was thought first to be a deformity is simply a minor variation that is "normal" for that particular patient. Inspection for deformity also includes documentation of any missing parts, such as loss of a fingertip or larger part from current or prior injury.

Aside from trauma, other problems that produce deformity include arthritis and inflammatory conditions, such as osteoarthritis, rheumatoid arthritis, psoriatic arthritis, lupus, and scleroderma. Tumors may produce deformity from mass effect.

Muscle *atrophy* also may be noted through careful inspection of the hand. Generalized atrophy may indicate disuse of the extremity, whereas atrophy of certain muscle groups may indicate specific nerve pathology. For example, long-standing carpal tunnel syndrome often results in atrophy of the thenar musculature. Ulnar nerve entrapment at the elbow may produce wasting of the interossei muscles, which in severe cases appears as deepened valleys between the metacarpals. Regional atrophy of subcutaneous fat may occur after local steroid injection.

Trophic changes in the hand are important observations to record, because they represent derangement of the sympathetic nervous system. Increased hair growth or altered sweat production (usually increased) may be signs of sympathetically mediated pain and are critical objective markers in making this difficult diagnosis.

Swelling is a common finding of disease or injury and can be identified by careful inspection and comparison with the uninvolved extremity. Localized swelling is a reliable clue to recent trauma or inflammation. Diffuse swelling is also an important finding because it is commonly caused by infection. Generalized swelling also can be indicative of a lymphatic or venous obstruction. Fractures as far proximal as the shoulder routinely result in a swollen hand within the first week after injury because of the effect of gravity on hematomas and traumatic exudates. Snug bandages or casts on the forearm also result in swollen fingers. Note that the dorsal subcutaneous space of the hand can accommodate a fair amount of edema fluid and is often the first area to show swelling, even if the trauma or infection is located on the palmar surface of the hand.

Inspection of the hand should also identify any wounds, skin abnormalities, or preexisting scars. The size and orientation of acute wounds should be carefully noted. The likelihood of nerve, artery, or tendon damage can often be predicted based on the location of the wound. Short, oblique lacerations just distal to the MCP joint of the fourth or fifth finger often result from fistfight injuries. When a clenched fist strikes another person in the mouth, the victim's tooth can easily cut through the skin of the assailant. This produces a relatively innocent looking laceration that actually represents penetration of the MCP joint capsule and bacterial inoculation of the joint.

Inspection for wounds also should include careful attention to the nail areas and web spaces for puncture sites or skin breakdown that can account for localized infections. Documentation of preexisting scars is important in clarifying any prior injuries or previous surgical treatments that might be relevant to the patient's current complaints.

The normal flexion creases of the hand and palm are useful reference points when describing the location of wounds or soft-tissue problems. Note that the position of these creases relative to the location of the underlying bone and joint can be misleading. For example, the MCP flexion crease is not situated over the

MCP joint itself, but actually is located over the mid-shaft of the proximal phalanx. The relative location of other skin creases is noted in the following (see "Normal Values").

PALPATION

Although the rest of the physical examination elements involve palpation, the process of touching the patient's extremity deserves its own category because it helps focus the remainder of the examination. This initial phase of palpation can be used to identify the following abnormalities:

Masses
Temperature abnormalities
Areas of tenderness
Crepitans
Clicking or snapping
Joint effusion

Although some growths or infections may produce a large enough mass to be seen easily on inspection, palpating the extremity often reveals masses that are not immediately obvious. Enlarged lymph nodes are often more easily felt than seen. Palpation may also demonstrate gross temperature differences between hands, possibly signaling an infectious, inflammatory, or vascular problem. Palpation may be the most useful in situations of trauma, whereby the examination and radiographic evaluation can be focused on those areas of the hand and wrist that are tender. Use of just one fingertip to carefully press on the bony prominences of the wrist and hand can be a remarkably sensitive diagnostic tool. Patients who present with a trigger finger, or tenosynovitis of the digital flexor tendons, often demonstrate tenderness and clicking when palpated over the distal palmar crease for the affected digit.

RANGE OF MOTION ASSESSMENT

Both passive and active motion should be carefully documented. Passive motion is demonstrated by holding the patient's finger or wrist and moving the joint in question without having the patient exert any muscular contraction. Active motion is that movement that occurs when the patient's own muscles contract. Passive motion yields information about joint stiffness owing to bony deformity or soft-tissue contractures. Active motion testing provides information regarding tendon continuity, nerve function, and muscular strength. Every finger joint can be independently tested and in many situations, active and passive motion should be documented for each joint. Aside from the amount of passive and active motion present, it is important to note whether motion causes any pain or is associated with instability or crepitans, as might be the case in situations of acute trauma, infection, or inflammation.

STABILITY ASSESSMENT

Stability testing often requires the examiner to use both hands, usually holding both proximal and distal to the joint in question, and then gently moving the joint passively to stress the ligaments that stabilize the joint. Loss of normal laxity is just as important a finding as too much laxity. Testing should also be done with the finger joints in positions of flexion and extension, because these different positions normally result in differing amounts of joint stability. For example, the true collateral ligaments of the MCP joints are tighter in flexion; therefore, passively flexing the MCP tightens the ligament and allows it to be tested when the joint is stressed side-to-side. A common ligament injury in the thumb is rupture of the ulnar collateral ligament of MCP (gamekeeper's thumb). Stressing the thumb MCP joint from side-to-side often makes this diagnosis (see "Special Tests").

The wrist joint is another area in which stability testing is important. The ligament connections between the different carpal bones should be carefully assessed, because instability of the wrist often leads to irregular load distributions and the development of posttraumatic arthritis. Palpation of the carpal bone prominences while the wrist is put through a passive range of motion often demonstrates instability patterns (see "Special Tests").

MUSCLE AND TENDON ASSESSMENT

The muscles and tendons that move the hand and wrist are divided into myotendinous units that have origins and insertions within the hand (intrinsic muscles) and myotendinous units that span the forearm and hand (extrinsic muscles). Both intrinsic muscle and extrinsic muscle groups can be divided into flexors and extensors. Although the ability to make a first and straighten up all the fingers offers general information about active range of motion, more detailed testing of individual muscles and tendons is often necessary. Evaluation of the muscles and tendons should consider both the integrity of the tendon and the strength of the muscle. In general, to test muscle strength you should "ask a muscle to do what it does" and then resist that motion. Muscle strength should be graded using a standard method (Table 1).

TABLE 1. *Grading the strength of muscle contractions*

Muscle grade	Physical examination findings
0	No contraction
1	Fibrillations or faintly palpable contraction
2	Muscular contraction that is insufficient to overcome the force of gravity
3	Muscular strength sufficient to overcome gravity through the full range of motion
4	Diminished strength on resistance testing
5	Normal strength

SPECIFIC TESTING OF CERTAIN MUSCLES

The flexor pollicis longus muscle inserts on the base of the distal phalanx of the thumb and can be tested by asking the patient to flex the distal joint of the thumb (Fig. 1). The flexor digitorum profundus tendon can be tested by asking the patient to flex the distal interphalangeal joint of the involved finger while the examiner blocks flexion of the proximal interphalangeal joint in the same finger and the flexor digitorum profundus function of adjacent fingers (Fig. 2). The flexor digitorum superficialis is tested by asking the patient to flex the proximal interphalangeal joint of only the involved finger. The other fingers must be blocked in extension to avoid interference from the flexor digitorum profundus of the finger being examined (Fig. 3). The flexor carpi ulnaris and flexor carpi radialis are tested by asking the patient to volar flex the wrist and then palpating the tendon or muscular contraction in its anatomic location.

The *first dorsal wrist compartment* contains the tendons of the *abductor pollicis longus (APL),* which inserts at the dorsal base of the thumb metacarpal, and the extensor pollicis brevis (EPB), which inserts at the dorsal base of the proximal phalanx of the thumb. These are evaluated by asking the patient to "bring

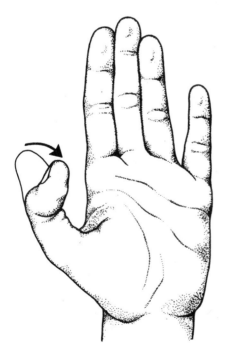

FIG. 1. Testing for flexor pollicis longus musculotendinous function.

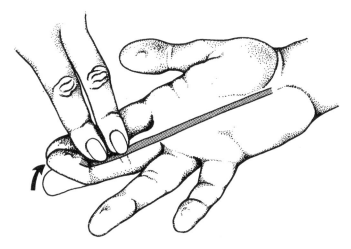

FIG. 2. Testing for flexor digitorum profundus musculotendinous function.

your thumb out to the side" (Fig. 4). The examiner can palpate the taut tendons over the radial side of the wrist going to the thumb.

The *second dorsal wrist compartment* contains the tendons of the *extensor carpi radialis longus (ECRL)* and the *extensor carpi radialis brevis (ECRB)* muscles (Fig. 5). They insert at the dorsal base of the index and middle metacarpals, respectively. These are evaluated by asking the patient to "make a

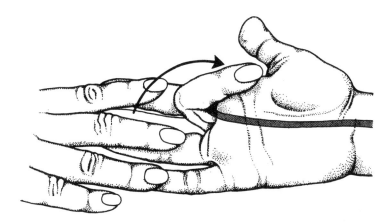

FIG. 3. Testing flexor digitorum superficialis musculotendinous function.

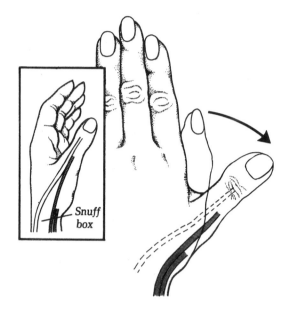

FIG. 4. Testing for extensor pollicis brevis and abductor pollicis longus musculotendinous function.

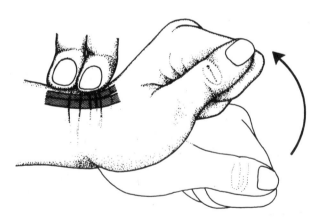

FIG. 5. Testing for extensor carpi radialis longus and extensor carpi radialis brevis musculotendinous function.

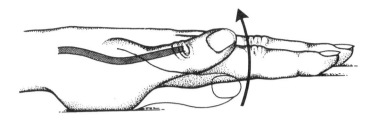

FIG. 6. Testing for extensor pollicis longus musculotendinous function.

fist and bring your wrist back strongly." The examiner can give resistance and palpate the tendons over the dorsoradial aspect of the wrist.

In the *third dorsal wrist compartment,* the *extensor pollicis longus (EPL)* tendon passes around Lister's tubercle of the radius and inserts on the dorsal base of the distal phalanx of the thumb. Placing the hand flat on the table and having the patient lift only the thumb off the surface evaluates this muscle (Fig. 6).

The *fourth dorsal wrist compartment* contains the tendons that are the MCP joint extensors of the fingers (Figs. 7 and 8). The *extensor digitorum communis (EDC)* and the *extensor indicis proprius (EIP)* muscle tendons are evaluated by asking the patient to "straighten your fingers" and observing MCP joint extension.

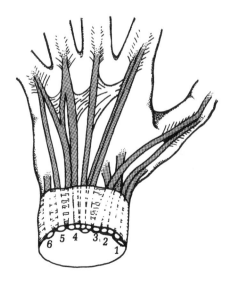

FIG. 7. Arrangement of extensor tendons at the wrist into six compartments: dorsal and cross-sectional views.

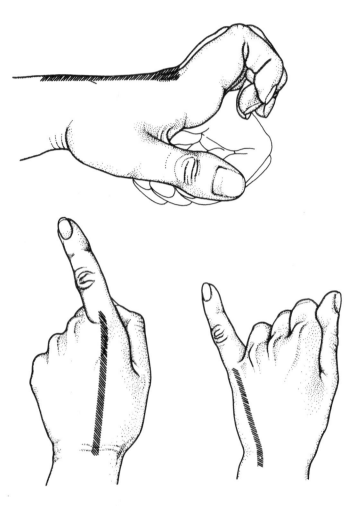

FIG. 8. Testing for extensor digitorum communis, extensor indicis proprius, and extensor digiti minimi musculotendinous function.

The EIP tendon can be isolated on examination by asking the patient to "bring your pointing finger out straight, with the other fingers bent in a fist." The EIP is acting alone to extend the index finger MCP joint (Fig. 8).

The *fifth dorsal wrist compartment* contains the tendon of the extensor digiti minimi (EDM) (Fig. 8). This is evaluated by asking the patient to "straighten out your small finger with your other fingers bent in a fist." This extends the MCP joint of the small finger. The EDM is acting alone to extend the small finger.

The *sixth dorsal wrist compartment* contains the tendon of the *extensor carpi ulnaris (ECU),* which inserts at the dorsal base of the fifth metacarpal (Fig. 9).

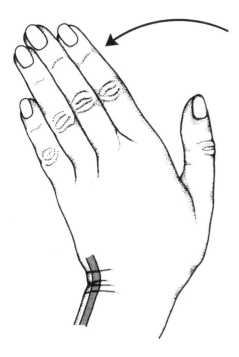

FIG. 9. Testing for extensor carpi ulnaris musculotendinous function.

This is evaluated by asking the patient to "pull your hand up and out to the side." The taut tendon can be palpated over the ulnar side of the wrist just distal to the ulnar head.

Extrinsic Extensor Tightness

The extensor tendons can become adherent over the dorsum of the hand or wrist, limiting finger flexion. Maintaining the wrist in neutral and passively extending the MCP joint and flexing the PIP joint can test this. Normally, the PIP joint should flex. The test is then repeated with the MCP joint passively flexed. If the PIP joint will passively flex when the MCP joint is extended, but will not flex readily with the MCP joint flexed, the adherent extrinsic extensors are check reining the simultaneous flexion of finger MCP and PIP joints. This is called "extrinsic extensor tightness."

INTRINSIC MUSCLES

The intrinsic muscles of the hand are those that have their origins and insertions within the hand. These are the thenar muscle groups, *adductor pollicis (AdP),* lumbrical, and interosseous muscles, and the hypothenar muscle group.

The Thenar Muscles

The thenar muscles are the muscles covering the thumb metacarpal. They are the *abductor pollicis brevis (APB), opponens pollicis (OP),* and *flexor pollicis brevis (FPB).* These muscles move the thumb into opposition (Fig. 2) and can be evaluated by asking the patient to "touch the thumb and small fingertips together so that the nails are parallel" (Fig. 10). They can also be tested by asking the patient to place the dorsum of the hand flat on the table and raise the thumb up straight to form a 90-degree angle with the palm (Fig. 2). It is helpful to examine and compare the contralateral hand in a similar way to detect slight variations in muscle mass and function. The motor branch of the median nerve usually innervates the thenar muscles. In some patients, however, the thenar muscles may be partially innervated by the ulnar nerve.

The Adductor Pollicis Muscle

Thumb adduction is separately tested by having the patient forcibly hold a piece of paper between the thumb and radial side of the index proximal phalanx

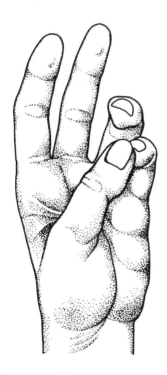

FIG. 10. Testing for thumb opposition.

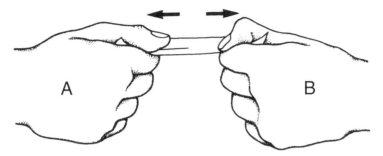

FIG. 11. Froment's sign is positive in hand B.

(Fig. 11). The muscle that powers this motion is the AdP, which is innervated by the ulnar nerve. When this muscle is weak or nonfunctioning, the thumb IP joint flexes with this maneuver (Froment's sign). In this evaluation the two hands must be compared.

The Interosseous and Lumbrical Muscles

The interosseous and lumbrical muscles act on the fingers to flex the MCP joints and extend the IP joints. The interosseous muscles also abduct and adduct the fingers. The ulnar nerve innervates the interosseous muscles, which lie on either side of the finger metacarpals. They can be evaluated by asking the patient to "spread your fingers apart" while the examiner palpates the first dorsal interosseous to see if it contracts. In another test, with the hand flat on a table, the patient is asked to elevate the middle finger (i.e., hyperextend the MCP joint with the IP joints straight) and radially and ulnarly deviate it (Fig. 12). (This eliminates the extrinsic extensors, which some patients can use to mimic interossei finger abduction-adduction.)

The Hypothenar Muscles

The hypothenar muscles—*abductor digiti minimi (ADM), flexor digiti minimi (FDM),* and *opponens digit minimi (ODM)*—are evaluated as a group by asking the patient to "bring the small finger away from the other fingers" (Fig. 13). This muscle mass can be palpated, and often a dimpling of the hypothenar skin is noted.

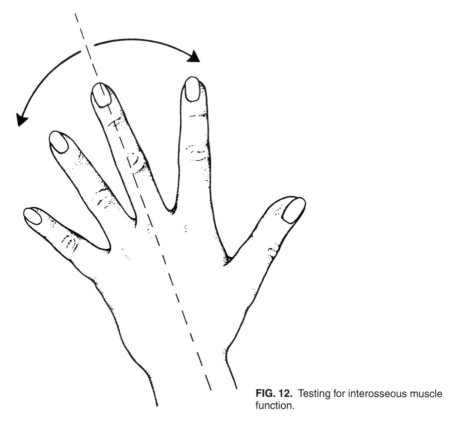

FIG. 12. Testing for interosseous muscle function.

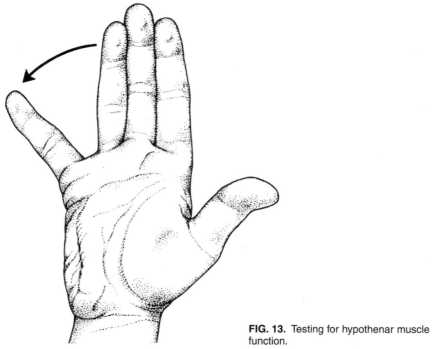

FIG. 13. Testing for hypothenar muscle function.

NERVE ASSESSMENT

Evaluation of the peripheral nerves should focus on motor and sensory function. The radial, median, and ulnar nerves must all be carefully assessed for motor function. Extension of the thumb IP joint is a good test of radial motor function. Palmar abduction of the thumb tests for the recurrent motor branch of the median nerve, whereas digital flexion of the thumb and index IP joints (the A-OK sign) tests for the anterior interosseous branch of the median nerve. Having the patient attempt to cross their fingers, which requires use of the interossei muscles, can assess ulnar nerve motor function. The strength of muscle function should also be evaluated in addition to noting the presence of motor function.

Sensibility testing also relies on knowledge of peripheral nerve anatomy. Radial nerve sensibility should be tested on the dorsal thumb-index web space. Median sensibility should be tested on the palmar surface of the index finger or thumb. Ulnar sensibility can be assessed accurately by testing the palmar aspect of the little finger. Individual digital nerve function should be evaluating by assessing both the radial and ulnar sides of each fingertip, on the palmar aspect.

Comprehensive sensibility evaluation should include light touch perception of the patient, and more sophisticated methods of assessment, such as static and dynamic two-point discrimination. Using a caliper, applied to the digit longitudinally, the smallest distance the patient can distinguish between the two points is measured. The two-point discrimination test is a very specific test for determining integrity of sensory nerve function. When examining digital nerve function, it is important to remember that each digit has a radial and ulnar digital nerve. Semmes-Weinstein monofilament testing and temperature testing also may be useful.

VASCULAR ASSESSMENT

Evaluation of blood supply to the hand and fingers relies on both inspection and palpation skills. As noted, arterial interruption often produces a white or grayish discoloration of the affected area, whereas venous blockage produces a congested, purple-blue color. Other clues to vascular abnormalities include temperature abnormalities (i.e., coolness) and loss of soft tissue pressure (abnormal turgor). Subungual splinter hemorrhages on the fingers may be a clue to the presence of proximal arterial lesion and embolic phenomena to the digits. Capillary refill is another way of assessing circulation. Pressing down on the fingertip or nail bed produces a localized area of white color, which, when pressure is released, should "refill" and turn pink within 2 seconds. Delay of refill longer than this may be an indicator of vascular insufficiency or poor digital turgor.

The Allen's test is helpful in determining whether there is independent supply of the hand by the radial or ulnar artery at the wrist. The examiner occludes both the radial and ulnar arteries at the wrist while the patient makes a tight fist to force blood out of the hand. The patient then opens the hand and the examiner releases pressure on one of the wrist vessels. If that particular vessel has an intact circulatory path for the hand, the palm and fingers should turn pink within 2 to

5 seconds. The test should then be repeated by releasing pressure on the other wrist vessel while occluding the first. Ulnar artery thrombosis, injury from a radial artery catheter, diabetic vascular disease, or an incomplete palmar vascular arch are all examples of problems that may produce an abnormal Allen's test.

Other findings associated with the vascular examination are associated pain, paresthesias, and paralysis. These problems are typically the product of ischemia and result when local tissue metabolic demands are not met by the available oxygen and nutrient supply.

SPECIAL TESTS

Palpation

Grind Test

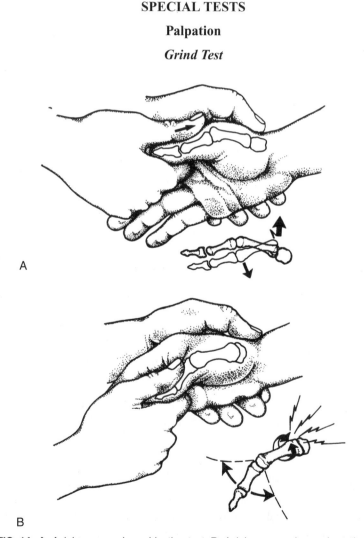

A

B

FIG. 14. A: Axial compression-adduction test. **B:** Axial compression and rotation test.

This is used to test for abnormalities at the thumb carpometacarpal joint (Fig. 14). The patient's wrist is held with the examiner's left hand and the thumb metacarpal is held with the examiner's right hand. The examiner then applies an axial load to the thumb metacarpal (pushing proximally) and gently rotates it side-to-side. Positive findings include significant pain, crepitans, and lateral subluxation of the metacarpal.

Finkelstein's Test

This is used to test for DeQuervain's tendinitis, or inflammation of the extensor and abductor tendons to the thumb (extensor pollicis longus and brevis, and abductor pollicis longus) (Fig. 15). The patient is asked to make a fist with the thumb under the other digits. The examiner then gently ulnarly deviates the wrist, which places great tension on the tendons in question. If these tendons are inflamed, the patient will report discomfort in the area of the first dorsal compartment.

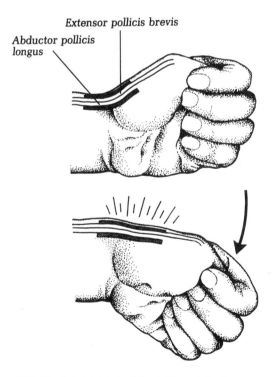

FIG. 15. Finkelstein's test for deQuervain's disease.

Range of Motion Assessment

Flexor Profundus Test

This is used to test continuity of the flexor digitorum profundus tendons (Fig. 2). Each finger is tested individually. The examiner places the patient's MCP and PIP joint in full extension and asks the patient to flex the tip of that finger. Active flexion at the DIP joint confirms that the flexor profundus is intact and that the muscle belly and corresponding motor nerve are functional. If the PIP joint is not held in flexion, the patient may bend the digit using the flexor sublimis tendon, and it can be confusing as to whether the profundus tendon is independently functional.

Flexor Sublimis Test

This is used to test continuity of the flexor digitorum sublimis tendon (Fig. 3). Each finger is tested individually. The examiner holds the patient's hand palm up on a flat surface, with the MCP, PIP, and DIP joints fully extended. The finger to be tested is then released and the patient is asked to flex it. The flexor profundus tendons are kept inactive with the DIP joints of the other fingers held in full extension, because the profundus muscles share a common origin. If one profundus is blocked from moving, all the profundus tendons cannot move; therefore, holding the DIP joints in extension isolates the flexor sublimis as the only mobile tendon. The patient will be able to flex the released finger only at the PIP joint, confirming that the flexor sublimis is intact.

BUNNEL'S TEST FOR INTRINSIC MUSCLE TIGHTNESS

To test for finger intrinsic muscle tightness the MCP joint of the finger is held in extension (0 degrees neutral position) while the examiner passively flexes the PIP joint (Fig. 16). The MCP joint is then flexed and the PIP joint is passively flexed in the same manner as before. If the PIP joint can be passively flexed with the MCP joint in flexion, but cannot be fully flexed when the MCP joint is extended, there is tightness of the intrinsic muscles. This is called "intrinsic tightness."

EXTRINSIC TIGHTNESS TEST

If the PIP joint can be easily flexed while the MCP joint is extended, but then becomes tight when the MCP joint is flexed, the patient is manifesting tightness of the extensor tendon ("extrinsic" tightness). If, however, passive PIP is easier with the MCP joint flexed than extended, the patient is demonstrating intrinsic tightness because of contracture of the lumbrical muscle.

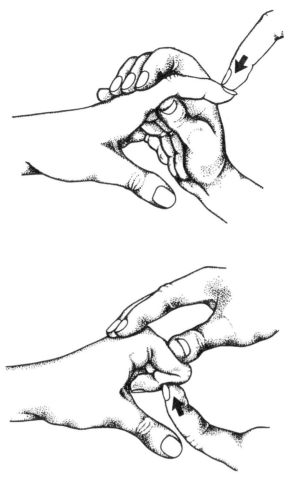

FIG. 16. Intrinsic muscle tightness.

Stability Assessment

Scaphoid Stability Test

This test is used to test for carpal ligament disruption between the scaphoid and lunate. The examiner's left hand is used to palpate the scaphoid's distal pole, which can be felt as a bony prominence on the palmar aspect of the wrist. The examiner then uses their right hand to gently move the wrist into radial and ulnar deviation. In radial deviation, the scaphoid moves into a position of relative flexion, and the distal pole can be felt to move into a position of more palmar prominence. With ulnar deviation of the wrist, the scaphoid assumes an extended position, and distal pole's prominence will diminish. If radial and ulnar deviation movements do not change the distal pole's position, then incompetence of the scaphoid ligament should be suspected. Other conditions affected the scaphoid, such as fracture nonunion or arthritis, may also produce fixed posture of the scaphoid (and possibly pain) with radial and ulnar deviation of the wrist.

Triquetrolunate Ballottement Text (LT Shear or Shuck Test)

This test is done to evaluate the patient for instability of the triquetrolunate ligament. The lunate is stabilized between the thumb and index finger of the examiner's nondominant hand with the wrist in a neutral position. The examiner pushes the triquetrum in a dorsal direction with the other hand. The test is positive if it reproduces the patient's pain or is unstable.

Midcarpal Instability Test

Most often these patients have pain on the ulnar side of the midcarpal row. The examiner stabilizes the distal radius and ulna with his nondominant hand starting with the wrist in radial deviation. The examiner moves the wrist into ulnar deviation. When the test is positive a "clunk" is felt on ulnar deviation as the midcarpal subluxation is reduced.

Ulnar Carpal Abutment Test

Patients with tears of the triangular fibrocartilage complex (TFCC) have pain on the ulnar side of the wrist. Often they also have a "clicking" with wrist deviation and forearm rotation. Palpate the wrist just distal to the ulna to test for general TFCC tenderness. The examiner stabilizes the wrist with his nondominant hand and moves the wrist into maximum ulnar deviation to perform the ulnar carpal abutment test. The test is positive if it reproduces the patient's pain or is associated with a significant click or pop.

Gamekeeper's Test

This is used to test for ulnar collateral ligament disruption at the thumb MCP joint (Fig. 17). The examiner holds the patient's thumb metacarpal with one hand, and the patient's thumb proximal phalanx with the other hand. With the patient's thumb MCP joint first fully extended, gentle radial deviation is applied to the thumb tip MCP joint, which stresses the ulnar collateral ligament. Tightness of the joint should be noted, and if the joint is lax, the examiner should note whether an endpoint is present. The same maneuver is then performed with the MCP joint held in about 30 degrees of flexion. Sometimes the ulnar collateral ligament can be disrupted and yet the patient's MCP joint does not feel unstable

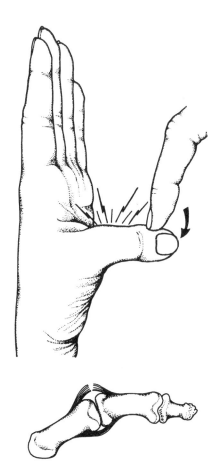

FIG. 17. Rupture of ulnar collateral ligament of the metacarpophalangeal joint of the thumb.

unless tested in both positions. The examiner should also test the patient's other thumb as a reference because there can be significant individual variation for collateral ligament tightness.

Nerve Assessment

Prune Test

This is used to test sensory nerve function in the fingers. The finger in question is held in a cup of water for about 5 to 10 minutes. Glabrous skin that has normal sensory innervation will wrinkle up (prune) after being submersed for this period of time. Sensory nerve interruption manifests itself as a finger that does not wrinkle despite prolonged immersion. This test can be particularly useful in evaluating sensibility in children or other patients who may not be able to volunteer sensibility information.

Tinel's Test

This is used as a provocative test for carpal tunnel syndrome (Fig. 18). The examiner percusses (with two fingers) over the distal palmar crease in the midline (over the pathway of the median nerve) with the patient's wrist in a position of supination. The test is considered positive (and suggestive of carpal tunnel syndrome) if the patient reports paresthesias in the median nerve distribution when the nerve is percussed.

Phalen's Test

This is also used as a provocative test for carpal tunnel syndrome (Fig. 19). The patient's wrist is held in a position of maximum flexion for up to 2 minutes.

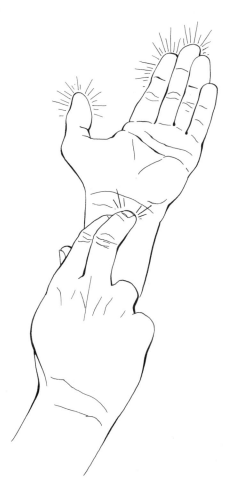

FIG. 18. Tinel's sign.

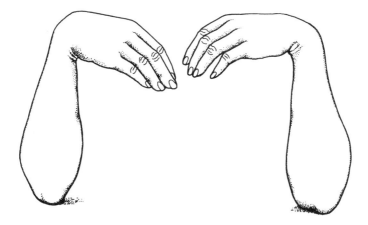

FIG. 19. Phalen's sign (wrist flexion test).

The test is considered positive if the patient reports paresthesias in the median nerve distribution.

Froment's Sign

This is used as a provocative test to assess for ulnar nerve related motor weakness (Fig. 11). The patient is asked to hold a piece of paper by grasping it between the thumb and index fingers in a side-to-side manner. The examiner then slowly pulls the paper away from the patient while encouraging him to hold on to it. If the ulnar nerve is functional and the first dorsal interosseous and thumb adductor muscles are strong, then the patient's thumb IP joint will remain extended. If there is weakness of the thumb adductor, then the patient will flex the thumb IP joint in order to compensate for the weakness. This is also sometimes referred to as Bunnel's "O" sign.

Jeanne's Sign

This is present when there is loss of lateral or key pinch of the thumb because of weakness or adductor pollicis muscle (owing to ulnar nerve dysfunction). When attempting a key pinch, patients demonstrate hyperextension of the thumb MCP joint.

Wartenberg's Sign

This is a finding that characterizes ulnar nerve-related motor weakness. The patient is asked to hold his fingers fully adducted with the MCP, PIP, and DIP joints fully extended. If the third palmar interosseous muscle is weak (usually because of ulnar nerve dysfunction), the force of the extensor digiti minimi tendon is unopposed and the small finger tends to deviate (abduct) away from the ring finger.

Threshold Tests

These modalities (e.g., von Frey pressure test with Semmes-Weinstein monofilament) test single nerve fibers that innervate a receptor. They are thought to be more sensitive than innervation density tests in determining early nerve damage. Another example of a threshold test is use of a variable amplitude vibrometer.

Innervation Density (Two-Point Discrimination)

These tests measure the innervation of multiple overlapping receptors, and as a result may remain almost normal even in the presence of advanced nerve pathology. Normal two-point discrimination at the fingertips is considered to be 6 mm or less.

Vascular Assessment

Allen's Test

Allen's test at the wrist (Fig. 20) is used to test ulnar and radial artery blood flow to the hand.

1. The patient makes a tight fist with his or her hand. This exsanguinates the hand of blood flow.
2. The examiner then occludes blood flow at both the radial and ulnar arteries by compressing these vessels at the patient's wrist.
3. The patient is then asked to gently open his or her fist and hold the fingers in a relaxed position (not hyperextension).
4. The examiner then releases the radial vessel while maintaining pressure on the ulnar vessel.
5. The time it takes for the hand and fingers to refill with blood is noted by observing how quickly the hand and fingers turn pink. Normal refill is considered within 5 seconds or less.
6. The entire process (steps one through four) is repeated, except this time the ulnar artery is released. Capillary refill time is noted again. Occlusion of the radial or ulnar artery because of thrombosis or disease is demonstrated by prolonged refill times. The Allen's test always should be performed prior to placement of a radial artery catheter, because placement of such a catheter often results in thrombosis of the radial artery. Radial artery catheter place-

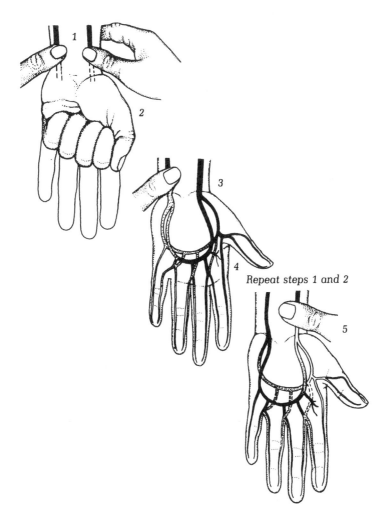

FIG. 20. Allen test for arterial patency.

ment can result in ischemic necrosis of the digits if the ulnar artery has pre-existing blockage.

Allen's test for the finger ("digital Allen's test") is used to assess digital arterial supply to the finger.

1. The patient fully flexes the finger to be tested and holds this position. This exsanguinates the finger.

2. The examiner then occludes both digital vessels by applying pressure at the base of the finger.
3. The patient is then asked to gently extend the finger and hold it in a relaxed position (not hyperextension).
4. The examiner then releases the radial vessel while maintaining pressure on the ulnar vessel.
5. The time it takes for the finger to refill is noted. A capillary refill time of less than 2 to 3 seconds is considered normal.
6. The entire process (steps 1 through 4) is repeated, except the ulnar artery is released this time. Again, capillary refill time is noted by observing how quickly the finger turns pink.

See Appendix 5 (Normal Values) for more information.

5

History and Physical Examination of the Child

The initial evaluation of a child with a congenital anomaly requires patience, empathy, knowledge, and a support staff. The conversation between doctor and family should be in lay terms with avoidance of medical jargon, except for important terminology concerning the named diagnosis. Misconceptions concerning the anomaly and its underlying pathogenesis are common and should be dispelled. Children with considerable anomalies or an underlying syndrome require medical, psychological, financial, and social assistance. This type of care is best provided at an institution familiar with the care of "challenged" children.

The history should be comprehensive and include questions concerning familial occurrence of limb anomalies, prenatal problems, birth history, and child development. The family history is particularly pertinent in congenital anomalies with known familial propagation, such as polydactyly and syndactyly. The prenatal history is important with regard to possible causes. Inquiry includes questions about previous pregnancies, stillbirths, or miscarriages. The birth history should include the duration of pregnancy, time and length of delivery, position at time of birth (e.g., breech presentation), and posture of the affected limb(s). Details about the achievement of developmental milestones (e.g., sitting, standing, walking, and talking) are important, because the presence of a congenital anomaly does not negate the possibility of additional problems, such as cerebral palsy.

Accurate diagnosis of limb anomalies also requires a basic knowledge of potential genetic and chromosomal causes to direct referral for genetic analysis and counseling. The role of the clinical geneticists is expanding and genetic testing for limb malformations is gradually increasing in its availability and clinical applicability. The child needs to be examined gradually and carefully without unnecessary handling. Age-appropriate toys and props are used during the examination and provide valuable information in terms of hand usage and dexterity. The examination can occur while a parent is holding the child, and playful activities can be incorporated into the evaluation.

49

The physical examination should include a complete musculoskeletal examination. The affected limb(s) are examined from hand to hemithorax and unilateral anomalies warrant careful inspection of the contralateral limb to ensure normality. Bilateral anomalies are often asymmetric and mild expression can exist unrecognized. In the newborn child, movement is difficult to elicit and primitive reflexes are employed to assess motion. The asymmetric tonic neck response, Moro reflex, and stimulation of palmar grasp are commonly employed. As the child ages, gross movement patterns and integration of the affected hand into functional activities are pertinent observations. Active range of motion measurements and manual muscle testing are not practical to assess in an infant or young child. Any other abnormalities, such as facial asymmetry, webbing, hairy patches, birthmarks, dimples, and abnormal genitals should be noted.

Following the initial evaluation, the physician may have a definitive diagnosis and sound understanding of the problem. An overall plan should be provided with realistic goals and expectations. In certain cases, the diagnosis and/or management are not straightforward or easily explainable. The physician should not be hesitant to elicit assistance from colleagues, experts, and published sources. Advances in technology have facilitated worldwide conferencing and appraisal. Digital photography allows capturing of valuable information that can be attached to electronic mail. The Internet has provided a readily accessible network for dissemination of cases to specialists in congenital hand surgery.

6

Anesthesia
for Hand Surgery

Adequate anesthesia is essential in the proper evaluation and treatment of most hand injuries. The type of anesthesia required is dictated by the level and severity of injury. Prior to administering any anesthetic, a careful neuromuscular examination of the area should be performed. The integrity of the sensory nerves and muscle–tendon units in the region to be anesthetized must be determined to assure these structures are not injured. Local anesthetics should not be given directly into an area that might be infected.

SELECTION OF ANESTHETIC AGENT

The most commonly used local anesthetic agents are lidocaine (1% or 2%) solution and bupivacaine (0.25% or 0.5%) solution. Lidocaine is effective quickly but lasts 1.5 to 3 hours. Bupivacaine is effective over 15 to 30 minutes, but lasts 3 to 10 hours. A 50-50 solution of the two agents is effective in combining the benefits of both agents. Solutions with epinephrine should not be used in blocks around the fingers and hand because of its vasoconstrictive effect. The maximum dose of anesthetic agents is lower when given without epinephrine. The maximum dose of lidocaine is 4.5 mg/kg. For adults, the maximum total dose should not exceed 300 mg. The maximum dose of bupivacaine is 2.5 mg/kg. The maximum total dose of bupivacaine should not exceed 175 mg. The addition of 1 mL of sodium bicarbonate solution per 10 mL of anesthetic alkalinizes the solution and decreases discomfort during injection. As with any injection, it is important to aspirate before injecting to avoid an intravascular injection of the agent. Early symptoms of toxicity from an intravascular injection include headache, ringing in the ears, numbness in the tongue and mouth, twitching of facial muscles, and restlessness. As the systemic levels of the agent increase, convulsions can result, followed by respiratory arrest and arrhythmias.

TYPES OF BLOCKS

Field Blocks

Direct infiltration into the wound edges is useful for many dorsal wounds and some palmar wounds where exploration of deep structures is not anticipated. It is also commonly used for procedures such as first dorsal compartment and trigger finger releases. When done with a long-acting anesthetic agent, it provides postoperative analgesia after short-acting anesthetics such as Bier blocks or general anesthesia. The technique is simple and may be converted to another type of block if insufficient. The disadvantage is that it makes the soft tissues edematous and sometimes hemorrhagic, thereby further injuring the soft tissue and distorting the anatomy.

When doing the block, a 25-gauge, 1½-in. needle is inserted at one end of wound and advanced parallel along one side of the incision. The anesthetic is injected subcutaneously until the wound edges are seen to swell. The deep spaces may be injected similarly if required.

Digital Blocks

Digital blocks are the preferred type of anesthesia for procedures done distal to the PIP joint. Caution should be used when giving digital blocks after injury to the digital artery that may require revascularization because the digital nerves and arteries run together. Digital blocks should also not be given when there is an infection around the MP joint.

A 25-gauge, 1½-in. needle is inserted distally in the web space where the skin innervation is less dense than in the palm (Fig. 1). The needle is advanced under the dorsal skin to the MP joint and 1 mL of anesthetic is injected into the subcutaneous space. The needle is withdrawn half way and directed palmarly between the MP joints. The needle is advanced until it is almost subcutaneous. Two to three milliliters are injected palmarly. The procedure is then repeated on the other side of the digit.

In the thumb, the two digital nerves are more palmar and closer together than in the digit. The ulnar digital nerve lies just palmar to the first web and the radial digital nerve lies just radial to the midline. Both nerves can be blocked by inserting the needle from ulnar to radial into the first web space at the MP joint. Two to three milliliters of anesthetic are injected transversely along the MP crease. Dorsal injections are given via sites at the radial and ulnar borders of the MP joint. Care should be taken to not give a "ring block," or circumferential injection at the MP joint. This block may tightly compress the tissues and compromise vascularity of the digit. As with any block in the hand, no effort is made to elicit paresthesias during the injection. The needle should be withdrawn and replaced in order to avoid injection into the nerve if paresthesias are elicited.

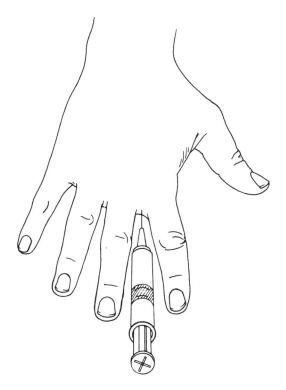

FIG. 1. Digital block.

Wrist Block

Four nerves may be blocked at the wrist. These are the median nerve, ulnar nerve, dorsal sensory branch of the radial nerve, and dorsal sensory branch of the ulnar nerve. The nerves to be blocked are dependent on the region of the hand that must be anesthetized. The thumb, index, middle, and radial border of the ring finger are innervated by the median nerve on the palmar surface and the dorsal sensory branch of the radial nerve on the dorsal surface. The small finger and the ulnar border of the ring finger are innervated by the ulnar nerve on the palmar surface and the dorsal sensory branch of the ulnar nerve on the dorsal surface. The median and ulnar nerves mainly innervate deep structures. In general, 5 mL of anesthetic are given at each site. Prior to injection, the patient should be told about the possibility of paresthesias if the nerve is punctured. The patient is told to tell the surgeon if any electric shocks are experienced. The anesthetic agent is injected only after the patient states no paresthesias are present. Once the injection begins, the needle should not be repositioned, thereby avoiding an intraneural injection of an anesthetized nerve.

The median nerve is located underneath the palmaris longus tendon. The injection is given ulnar to the palmaris longus tendon (Fig. 2A). A line is drawn from the ulnar border of the middle finger to the wrist crease if the patient does not have a palmaris longus tendon. With the wrist slightly extended, the needle is inserted just proximal to the wrist flexion crease and directed distally at a 30-

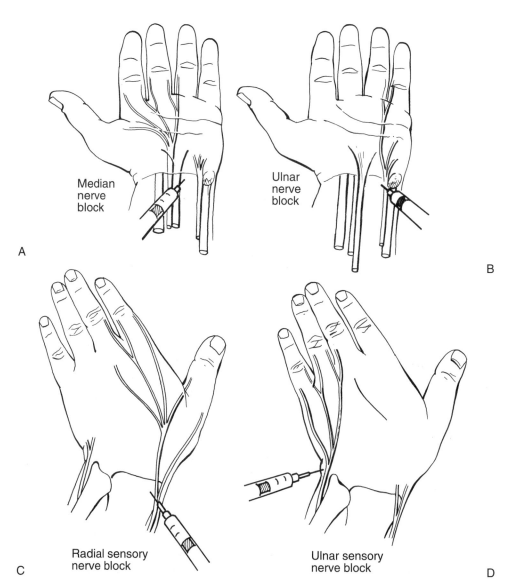

Median nerve block

Ulnar nerve block

A

B

Radial sensory nerve block

Ulnar sensory nerve block

C

D

FIG. 2. A: Median nerve block at the wrist. **B:** Ulnar nerve block at the wrist. **C:** Block of dorsal sensory branch of the radial nerve. **D:** Block of dorsal sensory branch of the ulnar nerve.

degree angle and slightly radially. Two distinct regions of resistance are felt as the needle is inserted. The first is on entering the skin and the second is piercing the antebrachial fascia. Once the patient states that no paresthesias are present, the solution is injected. A slight bulging in the palm, distal to the carpal tunnel, indicates proper placement of the agent.

The ulnar nerve lays ulnar to the ulnar artery in Guyon's canal. The neurovascular structures lie radial to the pisiform and ulnar to the hook of the hamate. The ulnar nerve is anesthetized by placing the needle at the radial border of the pisiform (Fig. 2B). The needle is inserted until it clears the radial edge of the pisiform and passes deep into Guyon's canal. Alternatively, the needle may be placed just radial to the flexor carpi ulnaris tendon at the wrist flexion creases. The solution is injected once the patient states that no paresthesias are present.

The dorsal sensory branch of the radial nerve exits from between the brachioradialis and extensor carpi radialis longus 5 to 8 cm proximal to the radial styloid. It divides into multiple branches distal to the radial styloid. The injection is placed 1 cm proximal to the radial styloid, radial to the radial artery (Fig. 2C). The needle is advanced dorsally to Lister's tubercle and 5 mL of anesthetic is subcutaneously administered throughout this region once the patient states that no paresthesias are present. Care is taken to aspirate before injecting to avoid an intravascular injection.

The dorsal sensory branch of the ulnar nerve passes from palmar to dorsal in the region of the ulnar styloid. The injection is placed at the level of the ulnar styloid beginning at the flexor carpi ulnaris, extending dorsally to the distal radioulnar joint (Fig. 2D). Five milliliters of anesthetic are administered subcutaneously throughout the region.

OTHER BLOCKS

The Bier block and the infraclavicular (axillary) block are two other commonly used blocks for the arm. Both are usually administered in a setting with resuscitation equipment available, preferably in a patient with an empty stomach because each of these blocks may have a complication with anesthetic toxicity. Many surgeons prefer that an anesthesiologist in an operating room perform these blocks.

A Bier block is an intravascular injection of an exsanguinated arm. Cast padding is applied to the arm and two 18- or 24-in. tourniquets are applied. An IV is inserted into a dorsal hand vein. The arm is exsanguinated by tightly wrapping it with an elastic bandage. Good exsanguination is the key to the procedure, obtaining both uniform anesthesia and a bloodless field. The distal tourniquet is first inflated to 250 or 100 mm Hg above the systolic blood pressure in hypertensive patients. The proximal tourniquet is then inflated and the distal cuff is released. Lidocaine 0.5% without preservatives is given as 3 mg/kg. The block is usually effective within 10 minutes. If the patient experiences tourniquet pain after 20 to 30 minutes, the distal cuff is inflated and the proximal cuff is then released, giving another 20 to 30 minutes of operative time. The tourniquet may be released 30 minutes after injection of the anesthetic.

The main advantage of Bier block anesthesia is that it is technically easy. Following release of the block, motor control returns in 10 to 15 minutes, allowing the surgeon to assess the results of a tenolysis. The disadvantages include tourniquet pain, which limits the usefulness of this block in procedures lasting more than 1 hour. The anesthetic effect lasts 5 to 10 minutes after release of the tourniquet, giving insufficient time for obtaining hemostasis and closing skin in some procedures. The block should not be used when infection or malignant tumors are present, as exsanguination of these limbs may spread the condition proximally. The major complication is early loss of tourniquet pressure, which is associated with systemic release of the agent and potential toxicity.

Infraclavicular blocks produce an effective sensory and motor blockade. With the use of long-acting anesthetics, these blocks also provide effective postoperative pain relief. The anesthetic agent is placed in the fascial compartment containing the peripheral nerves and axillary artery and vein. Considerable experience is required to adequately place this block and avoid an intravascular injection. The block is performed in a setting with resuscitation equipment available.

SELECTED REFERENCE

Ramamurthy S, Hickey R. Anesthesia. In Green DP, Hotchkiss RN, Pederson WC, eds. Operative hand surgery, 4th ed. Churchill Livingstone, New York, 1993, pp. 22–47.

7

Casting and Splinting

The purpose of a cast or splint is to immobilize the extremity in a desirable position to allow healing of the injured structures and to prevent late stiffness. Knowledge of the anatomy of the injured structures dictates the position of immobilization. Although no one dressing is right for all injuries, some general principles do apply.

Hand dressings should be comfortable and durable. They should be applied firmly enough to prevent them from slipping, but not so firmly as to impede circulation or increase edema. The dressing should immobilize the parts that need to be immobilized and permit freedom of motion of uninjured parts.

POSTOPERATIVE DRESSINGS

Placement of a proper postoperative dressing is an essential part of any operative hand procedure. Inattention to detail may compromise the results of the surgery. A hand dressing is applied in a series of layers, each with its own purpose.

The wound is covered with a single layer of a nonadherent dressing (Xeroform, Adaptec) (Fig. 1). Petroleum-impregnated gauze is removed more easily from the wound than dry gauze. A single layer is used to allow blood and serum to seep from the wound.

Over the nonadherent layer, opened 4 × 4 or 4 × 8 are placed around the wound to provide a bulky support (Fig. 2). The gauze draws fluid from the wound into the dressing. The gauze is placed where immobilization is needed. Opened gauze is placed in the web spaces to prevent maceration of the digits if the fingers and wrist are to be immobilized. Too much gauze, placed tightly into the webs, can compromise the circulation of an injured finger. No immobilization of the fingers is required and no dressings are placed in the webs if only the wrist needs to be immobilized.

For dressings that include the wrist, the next layer consists of large gauze, foam, or polyester fiber pads that are applied to the dorsal and palmar surfaces (Fig. 3). The purpose of this layer is to provide padding and draw fluid away from the wound. These pads are placed to immobilize the hand in the desirable position. The wrist is splinted in 30 to 40 degrees of wrist extension (Fig. 4). This is accomplished

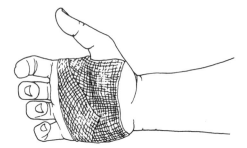

FIG. 1. Hand dressing: nonadherent gauze.

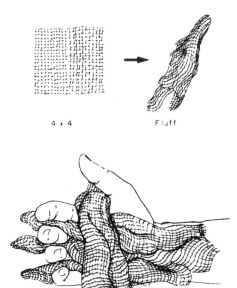

FIG. 2. Hand dressing: fluffy gauze.

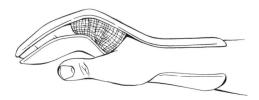

FIG. 3. Hand dressing: bulky adherent gauze.

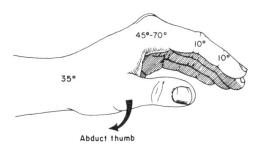

FIG. 4. Hand dressing: position of fingers.

by aligning the long axis of the thumb with the long axis of the forearm. When the fingers also need to be immobilized in the dressing, the metaphalangeal (MP) joints are flexed 60 to 70 degrees and the interphalangeal (IP) joints are held in 10 to 15 degrees of flexion. The collateral ligaments of the MP joints are on stretch in flexion and the IP joints in extension. Failure to position the joints properly in the dressing may lead to a contracture. The thumb is positioned in abduction at the carpometacarpal (CMC) joint and extension at the MP and IP joints. The pads are held in place with circumferential roller gauze. Gentle pressure is used in applying the roller gauze to keep the pads snug to the wound, but not constrict the hand.

Finally, a plaster or fiberglass splint is applied to keep the soft dressing in the desirable position (Fig. 5). Splints are used rather than casts for postoperative dressings and after reduction of fractures and dislocations in order to avoid a circumferential hard layer that might lead to constriction with swelling. Plaster is used more commonly because it is cheaper and easier to mold. Ten layers of plaster are placed on the palmar surface to immobilize only the parts that require immobilization. A dorsal splint may augment a palmar one on occasion. Care should be taken that cast padding extends at least 1 cm past the splinting material to prevent contact between the skin and plaster. The plaster is held in place with a bias-cut stockinette or a loosely placed Ace bandage. The surgeon holds the hand in the desirable position while the plaster hardens.

A sugar tong splint (Fig. 6) is a specific splint that is used to allow elbow flexion and extension while immobilizing forearm rotation and wrist motion. The hand, forearm, and elbow are padded with 3-ply of cast padding. Next, 10-ply of 3-in. plaster is placed from the palm of the hand up the volar forearm around the elbow and down the dorsum of the forearm finishing at the distal end of the metacarpals. The splint is molded and finished with a 3-in. gauze and ace wrap.

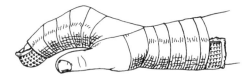

FIG. 5. Hand dressing: splint.

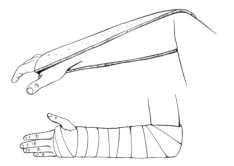

FIG. 6. A sugar tong splint is used to immobilize the carpus and forearm.

A finger dressing may be applied when the digit is injured and the immobilization does not need to extend proximally. Quite commonly, dressings are required for fingertip injuries. The wound is first covered with nonadherent gauze (Xeroform, Adaptec). A single 4 × 4 is cut one-third of the way from one edge for two-thirds of its distance parallel to that edge (Fig. 7A). The narrow strip is placed over the fingertip from the dorsal to palmar surface (Fig. 7B). The wide end is then wrapped around the fingertip (Fig. 7C). The excess is folded over the tip (Fig. 7D). The gauze is then held in place with 2-in. roller gauze, wrapped once around the wrist to hold it in place. The patient is instructed to report signs of tightness, such as throbbing pain or numbness after the block wears off because the fingertip cannot be observed.

Children are more likely to remove postoperative dressings than adults are; therefore, the younger the child the larger the dressing needed to protect the wound and immobilize the injured part. A long-arm dressing with a long-arm splint is required in children up to ages 2 to 3 years. A Velpeau dressing, holding the arm against the body, further protects the dressing (Fig. 8). The Velpeau dressing is made with a 3-in. stockinette. A piece approximately 2 ft long is longitudinally split for one-half of its distance. From the split side, the stockinette is placed over the arm to the axilla. The two split tails are passed around the back, one coming over the shoulder and one under the axilla. The two tails are tied, with care taken not to compress the contents of the axilla. A small hole is made in the stockinette just distal to the fingertips. The tails are passed through the hole and again tied. The fingertips can be observed through the distal hole.

The last component of any postoperative dressing is a method of elevation. Elevation decreases postoperative swelling and pain, thereby promoting early mobilization of the hand. The hand should be placed above the level of the heart. The hand should always be higher than the elbow. The easiest way to do this is to place a sling, positioned so the hand is in the proper position. The patient should be reminded to frequently remove the sling for range of motion exercises of the shoulder and elbow. The hand should be placed on pillows when the patient is sitting. At night, a pillow may be wrapped around the hand with masking tape, which keeps it from falling into a dependent position. Elevation is required for the first few days to a week in most instances.

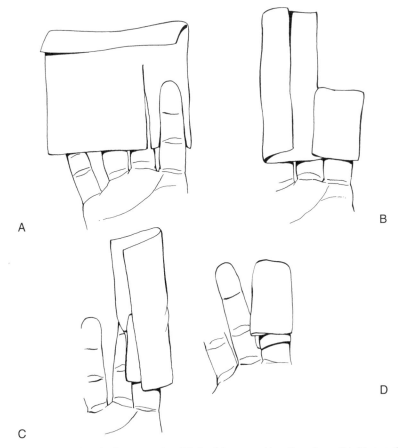

A

B

C

D

FIG. 7. Finger dressing. **A:** Cut gauze two-thirds of the way at junction of one-third to two-thirds. **B:** Wrap narrow end over fingertip from dorsal to palmar. **C:** Wrap wide end around finger. **D:** Fold excess over tip.

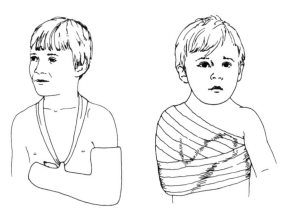

FIG. 8. Velpeau dressing.

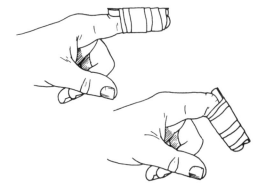

FIG. 9. Static splint for mallet finger.

SPLINTS

Splints are removable devices that are carefully fitted for a specific reason. The splint must be changed to meet the changing need of the healing tissues of the hand.

There are four types of splints. Static splints are rigid devices that maintain the hand in one position. This is the type most commonly applied following injuries. They are usually used during the immobilization phase to allow healing, decrease inflammation, and provide protection. An example is a palmar extension splint applied to the distal interphalangeal (DIP) joint for treatment of a mallet finger (Fig. 9).

Serial-static splints are rigid devices that are changed frequently to provide slow, progressive mobilization. They are most effective when remobilizing long-standing, mature scar. In the treatment of chronic boutonnière deformities, a palmar proximal interphalangeal (PIP) extension splint with a dorsal strap over the PIP joint is tightened and loosened frequently to stretch the flexion contracture (Fig. 10).

Dynamic splints have a rigid base and apply tension with springs, rubber bands, or coils. They provide a constant gentle force over a prolonged period of time. This type of splint is used during the proliferative stage of healing, rather than after the scar has matured. An example is a spring-loaded PIP extension splint placed after the development of a flexion contracture (Fig. 11).

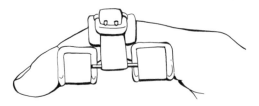

FIG. 10. Progressive static splint for boutonnière.

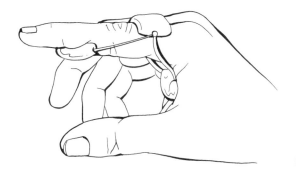

FIG. 11. Dynamic splint.

Semiflexible splints are made of a flexible material or have hinges. They allow a limited range of motion. A neoprene thumb spica splint is preferred by some patients over a static thumb spica splint to partially immobilize an arthritic CMC joint.

CASTS

Casts provide more rigid immobilization than splints. After cleansing the skin, 3-ply padding is applied to the hand and arm prior to cast application. Plaster casts can be molded into specific positions to stabilize specific injuries. By their nature, casts cannot be removed easily and may be more effective than splints in the unreliable patient.

There are four types of casts that are used most commonly in the upper extremity.

A short-arm cast extends from just proximal to the MP joints to 1 to 2 in. distal to the antecubital fossa. Care is taken to limit the plaster or fiberglass distally to allow full MP flexion, especially at the small finger. A short-arm cast immobilizes the distal radius and ulna, wrist, and proximal metacarpals. It is applied for stable distal radius fractures, capsular avulsion fractures of the wrist, dorsal triquetral fractures, and proximal metacarpal fractures.

A long-arm cast extends from just proximal to the MP joints to the mid-humerus. In most instances, the elbow is in 90 degrees of flexion and the forearm is in neutral rotation. Long-arm casts are used to limit motion at the distal radio–ulnar joint in addition to the wrist joint. It is used for unstable distal radius fractures, both bone forearm fractures, and unstable distal radioulnar joint injuries.

A thumb spica cast includes the thumb metacarpal. The IP joint may be included or excluded, depending on the injury. Long-arm thumb spica casts are used in the initial treatment of scaphoid fractures. Short-arm thumb spica casts are used for stable scaphoid fractures and thumb fractures. The IP joint is included in the initial treatment of injury to the ulnar collateral ligament of the MP joint of the thumb (gamekeeper's thumb) and proximal phalangeal fractures.

An intrinsic-plus cast is a short-arm cast with the plaster extending distally onto the fingers. The fingers are immobilized at 60 to 70 degrees at the MP joint and 10 to 15 degrees at the IP joint. Both the injured and neighboring fingers are included in the cast. This type of cast is used to treat fractures of the fingers. An intrinsic-plus cast of the ring and small fingers is placed for a fracture of the metacarpal neck of the small finger (boxer's fracture).

SELECTED REFERENCES

American Society for Surgery of the Hand, ed. Hand splinting. In 1998 Regional review courses in hand surgery. American Society for Surgery of the Hand, Rosemont, IL, 1998, pp. 18-1–18-7.

8

Distal Radius Fractures

GENERAL INFORMATION

Fractures of the distal radius are the most common group of fractures seen. These fractures represent a very heterogeneous group of injuries seen in a wide variety of clinical settings and age groups. Although common, management of some of these fractures may be controversial and challenging. Osteoporosis is a significant predisposing factor for the occurrence of the distal radius fractures after a minor injury and may also be a significant factor to be considered in the management of these injuries.

DIAGNOSTIC CRITERIA

The diagnosis of distal radius fractures is based on history and physical examination. X-rays are used to confirm the diagnosis. On rare occasions confirmation of a clinically suspected fracture may require imaging beyond plain x-rays (bone scan, a computed tomography [CT] scan, or a magnetic resonance imaging [MRI] scan).

History

Distal radius fractures most commonly occur as a result of excessive loading of the wrist in extension but may occur secondary to excessive loading in flexion, axial load, a shearing mechanism, or as a result of a direct blow. This may occur in a wide variety of clinical settings and represent low-, medium-, and high-energy injuries. The most common mechanism is a fall on an outstretched hand. Higher-energy injuries may occur as a result of a motor vehicle accident, a fall from a height, a sporting event, or an industrial injury.

These injuries are seen in all decades of life. Osteoporosis is a significant predisposing factor in elderly persons. A simple fall, which may result in no bony injury in a normal individual, may result in a distal radius fracture in an osteoporotic individual. Generally, a higher-energy mechanism of injury is required to induce a distal radius fracture between the second and sixth decade of life. There is a significant predominance of distal radius fractures in women beyond the sixth decade because of the prevalence of osteoporosis in this population.

Physical Examination

A wide spectrum of physical findings may be encountered because of the wide variation in clinical settings in which distal radius fractures are seen. Invariably, tenderness is present when the distal radius is palpated. Swelling may be quite mild in a low-energy nondisplaced fracture. In high-energy fractures, swelling may be so severe as to arouse suspicion of an acute carpal tunnel syndrome or compartment syndrome. Deformity of the affected wrist and hand may be present with a displaced fracture. Most commonly this will take the form of the so-called "silver fork deformity" (Fig. 1).

Skin integrity must be evaluated carefully. Abrasions from an associated fall are common. Although open fractures of distal radius are most commonly seen in a high-energy injury, open fractures also may be seen following a relatively simple fall in an osteoporotic individual in which significant fracture displacement combined with thin fragile integument result in a Grade 1 open injury.

Appropriate assessment of the neurovascular status of the involved extremity is essential. Median nerve compromise is not uncommon because of the high-energy nature of some of these fractures, as well as the marked displacement that may occur. Sensory and motor assessment of the median and ulnar nerves should be performed. If the examination is abnormal, then reassessment should be done following reduction of the fracture. Vascular compromise may occur as result of these injuries as well. Arterial laceration may occur from the sharp edge of the fracture, especially when severe dorsal displacement of the distal segment occurs. Venous compromise may occur as a result of a markedly displaced position and/or severe swelling. Ongoing assessment of neurovascular status may be necessary in higher-energy injuries, especially following reduction and plaster immobilization.

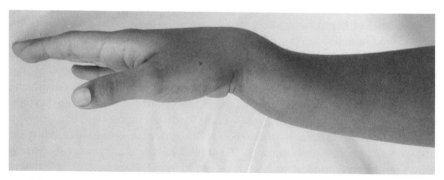

FIG. 1. A fall on an outstretched hand may result in a dorsal displacement of the distal radius. This characteristic appearance is known as the silver fork deformity.

Radiographic Assessment

Radiographic evaluation of the injured wrist is necessary to confirm the diagnosis of a distal radius fracture. Standard AP and lateral radiographs usually are sufficient to make the diagnosis. Additional oblique views sometimes are helpful in detecting a subtle nondisplaced fracture.

Accurate description of the fracture may be difficult. Historically, various patterns of distal radius fractures have been described using eponemonic nomenclature (Colle's fracture, Smith's fracture, Barton's fracture, etc.). More recently, numerous classification systems have been proposed; however, universal acceptance of any of these systems has not occurred because of a variety of shortcomings. It is essential that a clear and accurate description of the fracture can be made because of the heterogeneity of these fractures. It is important that these fractures are described in terms of displacement, comminution, and the radiographic parameters of articular surface tilt, radial length, radial inclination, and intraarticular extension (evaluating step-off and gapping of the articular surface) (Fig. 2). In order to accurately describe these parameters it is essential that a *true* AP and a *true* lateral radiograph be obtained.

A bone scan or MRI may be helpful in establishing the diagnosis on rare occasions when clinical suspicion suggests a distal radius fracture but radiographs do not reveal a fracture. Occasionally, a CT scan of the distal radius may be helpful in more accurately evaluating the articular surface for step off and gapping, as well as preoperative planning.

TREATMENT

Although the treatment options for all distal radius fractures are the same, selection of the most appropriate option should be individualized to the patient and the fracture. Treatment options include splinting, casting, closed reduction and casting, percutaneous pinning, external fixation, open reduction/internal fixation (ORIF), and combinations of these options. Generally, distal radius fractures require 6 weeks of immobilization to achieve satisfactory healing. This period of time may be shorter for patients under the age of 10 or longer for more complex fractures.

Nonunion of a fracture of the distal radius is rare. Malunion is much more common. The goal of distal radius fracture management is to achieve union of the fracture in as nearly an anatomic position as possible. Generally, there is a correlation between fracture outcome (motion, strength, and pain) and maintenance or restoration of normal or near normal distal radius morphology; however, because of the wide demographic distribution and spectrum of injury in these fractures, there may be significant variation in this correlation between outcome and morphology. In general, the more active and more significant demands an individual places on the injured wrist the more this correlation holds

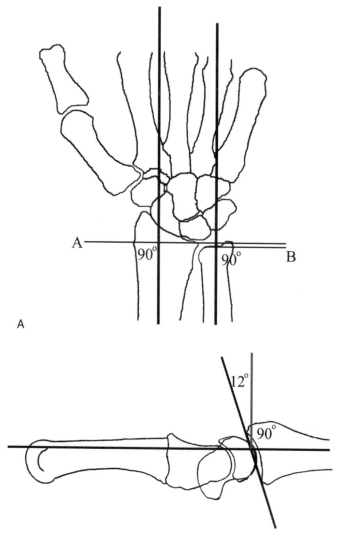

FIG. 2. A: Radial length is a measure of the degree of shortening of the ulnar side of the distal radius relative to the ulna. It is measured by taking the difference between two lines *A* and *B*. Line *A* is perpendicular to the long axis of the radius and contacts the distal ulnar margin of the radial articular surface. The second line, *B,* is drawn perpendicular to the long axis of the ulna and contacts the distal articular surface of the ulna. When radial length is not maintained (line *A* is proximal to line *B*), the ulna may impact on the carpus. **B:** Radial tilt represents a measure of the inclination of the articular surface of the radius seen on the lateral view. It represents the angle between a line contacting the dorsal and volar lips of the radius and a line perpendicular to the long axia of the radius. The normal tilt is approximately 12 degrees in a volar direction. Following a distal radius fracture the articular surface may be tilted back and expressed as dorsal tilt (as measured from the perpendicular).

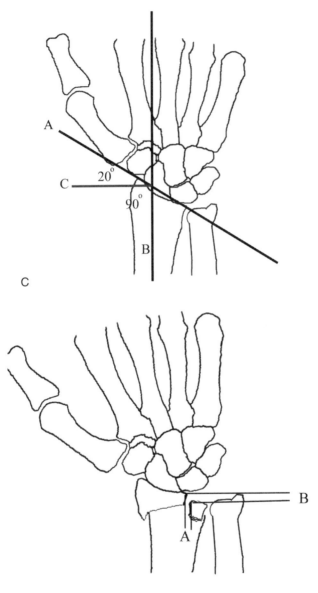

FIG. 2. *Continued.* **C:** Radial inclination represents the angle between a line contacting the distal edge of the radial and ulnar articular surfaces of the distal radius *(A)* and the perpendicular *(C)* to the longitudinal axis of the radius *(B)*. This normally measures approximately 20 and is frequently decreased following a distal radius fracture. **D:** Articular congruity is an important predictor of outcome of fractures of the distal radius with articular involvement. Both articular gapping *(A)* and articular depression or step-off *(B)* should be noted.

true. Skeletally immature individuals with significant capacity for remodeling and sedentary elderly individuals may be an exception to this rule.

Most nondisplaced fractures may be managed in a short arm cast or removable splint. The splint may be removed for hygiene purposes only; however, gentle active range of motion exercises may be initiated after approximately 4 weeks. These fractures should be reevaluated radiographically at approximately 1 week after initiation of treatment to verify that no displacement has occurred. Generally following 6 weeks of protection patients may progressively increase their activity. Hand therapy is usually unnecessary; however, maximum functional recovery may not occur for 6 months or longer.

Treatment of displaced fractures may be more challenging. In general, initial treatment requires closed reduction and splinting. A hematoma block (local anesthetic injected directly into the fracture site) and/or intravenous sedation facilitates closed reduction. Initially, most fractures are immobilized in a sugar tong splint. If postreduction radiographs demonstrate restoration of distal radius morphology, then nonoperative treatment in a cast should be recommended. The patient will need to be reevaluated at weekly intervals to ensure that the immobilization splint fits well and the reduction has been maintained. If satisfactory reduction has been maintained for 3 weeks, then it is unlikely that reduction will be lost. These fractures are often treated to union in a short arm cast. Maximum functional recovery may take 6 to 12 months.

If there is unsatisfactory restoration of distal radius morphology following an adequate attempt at closed reduction, or satisfactory reduction is not maintained, then the patient should be considered for operative treatment. It is important to evaluate each individual patient and their needs in making such a decision. Selection of specific operative treatment option(s) should be determined by consideration of the patient, fracture, and experience of the surgeon. Generally, hand therapy is initiated shortly after surgical treatment.

KEY POINTS

- Although common, this group of fractures remains one of the most challenging in terms of obtaining a consistently good outcome.
- Initiation of early active and passive range of motion (ROM) finger exercises is essential to good fracture outcome, and recognition of limited finger motion requires initiation of formal hand therapy at any point in the management of these fractures.
- Early mobilization of the shoulder may prevent the secondary development of rotator cuff tendonitis and adhesive capsulitis owing to limited shoulder use during fracture healing.
- Late (6 to 10 weeks postinjury) rupture of the extensor pollicis longus (EPL) tendon may occasionally occur, but is more characteristic of nondisplaced than displaced fractures.
- Initial immobilization is usually a sugar tong-type splint or widely split cast.

9

Carpal Fractures

SCAPHOID

General Information

The scaphoid is the most commonly fractured carpal bone. This fracture occurs most frequently in young adult men, but may be seen in elderly persons and patients as young as 12.

Diagnostic Criteria

The criteria for diagnosis of a scaphoid fracture include an appropriate history, clinical suspicion, and objective documentation (x-rays or other imaging modality) of the fracture. The consequences of undertreatment of a scaphoid fracture and over immobilization of a wrist sprain make it essential to conclusively determine that a scaphoid fracture either does or does not exist. The determination that a fracture is not present may be accomplished either by clinical examination (no tenderness in the snuffbox or over the distal pole of scaphoid) or imaging modalities (a negative plain x-ray is not conclusive). Failure to diagnosis a scaphoid fracture may lead to the development of nonunion and wrist arthritis. Other traumatic conditions producing wrist pain similar to that produced by a scaphoid fracture include distal radius fracture, fracture of another carpal bone, ligamentous injury to the wrist, and wrist sprain. A patient with a long-standing nonunion (who may be unable to recall any prior significant trauma to the wrist) may present with a more recent injury, which may lead to the incorrect conclusion that the fracture seen on x-rays is an acute injury.

History

Typically, a scaphoid fracture occurs as a result of a forceful extension of the wrist. Most commonly, this occurs as a result of a fall, motor vehicle accident, or sporting event mishap. The patient complains of pain on the radial aspect of the wrist, limited mobility, and some degree of swelling. It is not unusual for the patient to present for evaluation days and sometimes weeks after the injury. The patient may attribute his or her symptoms to a sprain or less severe injury to the wrist.

Physical Examination

Clinical examination should include observation for areas of swelling (commonly noted on the dorsal/radial aspect of the carpus) and ecchymosis (more commonly noted volarly). Palpation should include all areas of the wrist, including the distal radius and ulna, the anatomic snuffbox, the individual carpal bones, as well as the carpal metacarpal joints. Tenderness to palpation of the anatomic snuffbox or over the distal pole of the scaphoid should make a fracture of the scaphoid a diagnostic consideration. Wrist motion is usually reduced, but if there has been a delay between the injury and time of presentation, motion may be good.

Radiographic Assessment

Standard anterior posterior (AP) and lateral x-rays of the injured wrist should be obtained. In addition, a scaphoid view or an ulnarly deviated AP view is extremely helpful in producing a longitudinal view of the scaphoid and may help define a subtle, nondisplaced fracture. Fractures of the scaphoid may be seen in the proximal, middle, or distal third of the bone (Fig. 1). They may be described as nondisplaced, displaced, angulated, malrotated, and/or comminuted. The plain x-rays also should be inspected for evidence of degenerative changes secondary to a chronic nonunion (beaking of the radial styloid or narrowing of the radio-scaphoid joint space distal to the nonunion site) (Fig. 2).

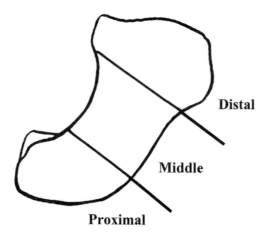

FIG. 1. Fractures of the scaphoid are classified as involving the proximal, middle (waist), or distal third (including scaphoid tubercle).

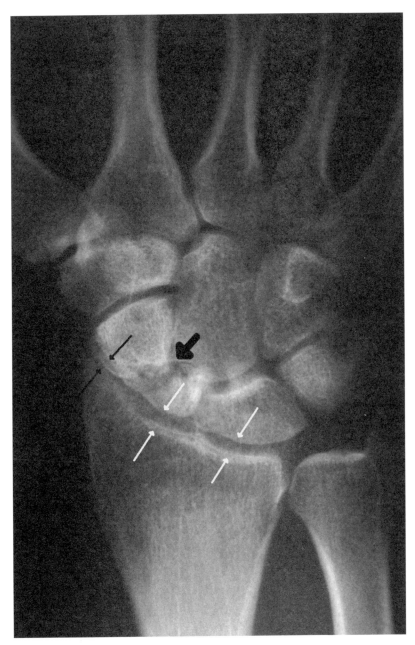

FIG. 2. A scaphoid nonunion may be difficult to distinguish from a fracture at times; however, the presence of a beaked appearance to the radial styloid and narrowing of the radioscaphoid joint *(small black arrows)* distal to the fracture nonunion site *(large black arrow)* all indicate that this is a nonunion and not an acute fracture. Note the radiocarpal joint space is well maintained *(white arrows)* proximal to the nonunion site.

Commonly, an acute fracture may not be seen on initial films. Repeat films taken in 10 to 14 days may subsequently reveal a fracture as a result of slight resorption of bone around the fracture site. If clinical suspicion suggests that a fracture still may be present in spite of negative delayed x-rays, further imaging studies are indicated. A bone scan, computed tomography (CT) scan, and magnetic resonance imaging (MRI) have all been reported to have a high level of sensitivity for detecting occult scaphoid fractures.

Treatment

The patient should be immobilized in a thumb spica splint if he or she presents with an acute injury and is clinically suspected to have a scaphoid fracture but no fracture is identified on x-rays. The patient should be discouraged from using the hand for any heavy activities.

Once the diagnosis of scaphoid fracture is made, treatment is dictated by the location of the fracture within the scaphoid as well as the degree of displacement of the fracture.

Fractures of the Middle Third (Waist)

Nondisplaced fractures of the waist of the scaphoid are the most common type of scaphoid fracture and should be immobilized in a thumb spica cast until radiographic evidence of healing is present. This typically takes between 9 and 12 weeks; however, it may take 16 weeks or longer. There is some evidence that the rate of union is slightly higher if a long arm thumb spica cast is used initially. The time to union also may be slightly shorter if a long-arm cast is used.

Fractures of the waist demonstrating more than 1 mm of displacement, comminution, angulation, or malrotation are at increased risk for the development of nonunion when treated with casting alone; therefore, operative treatment with open reduction and internal fixation generally is recommended for these fractures.

Fractures of the Proximal Third

Fractures of the proximal third of the scaphoid are also at increased risk for the development of non-union. Open reduction and internal fixation from a dorsal approach is generally recommended for these fractures.

Fractures of the Distal Third

Fractures of the distal third of the scaphoid generally heal more quickly and require a shorter period of immobilization. Unless a distal third fracture involves a significant portion of the distal pole articular surface and demonstrates more than 2 mm of step off, treatment in a short-arm thumb spica cast is recommended. The duration of treatment is generally 6 to 8 weeks, but must be correlated with clinical evaluation and the absence of tenderness at the fracture site. Rarely, a displaced intraarticular fracture of the distal pole may require open reduction internal fixation.

Aftercare

The type and location of the scaphoid fracture and the method of treatment determine aftercare. Once immobilization is completed, subsequent care may consist entirely of a home exercise program or require a formal course of hand therapy. Typically, this is determined on an individual basis. Generally, therapy is indicated following operative treatment. This may be initiated in the early postoperative period if rigid fixation is obtained.

Key Points

- Clinical suspicion is the key to appropriate diagnosis of scaphoid fractures.
- One should suspect a preexisting nonunion if the fracture appears too obvious.
- Operative treatment of nondisplaced waist fractures may be indicated in certain circumstances.

HOOK OF HAMATE

Diagnostic Criteria

Diagnosis of a fracture of the hook of the hamate usually requires a clinical index of suspicion and documentation of the fracture on an imaging study. Additional imaging studies are frequently needed to confirm the diagnosis because radiographic demonstration of the fracture may be difficult. Other considerations in the differential diagnosis of hypothenar hand pain may include contusion, sprain, fracture of another carpal bone, ulnar-sided carpal instability, hypothenar hammer syndrome, ganglion, and ulnar tunnel syndrome. Fracture of the hook of the hamate is distinguished from these other conditions by the presence of localized point tenderness and radiographic identification of the fracture or nonunion.

History

Fractures of the hook of the hamate frequently present in a subacute fashion or as an established nonunion. A history of an injury to the palmar surface of the hand frequently can be elicited. This may occur as the result of a fall onto the palmar surface of the hand or an atypical blow to the palm of the hand during participation in a club or racket sport (golf, tennis, baseball, etc.). The patient may complain of pain in the hypothenar region of the hand associated with direct pressure or loading as well as with forceful gripping or grasping with the fourth and fifth digits.

Physical Examination

Hypothenar swelling and/or ecchymosis may be present in the acute setting. Little or no restriction of motion is noted in both acute and delayed presentation. Point tenderness is noted with palpation of the palm over the hook of the hamate (Fig. 3). Pain may also be reproduced with attempted opposition of the small finger or resisted flexion of the ring and small fingers.

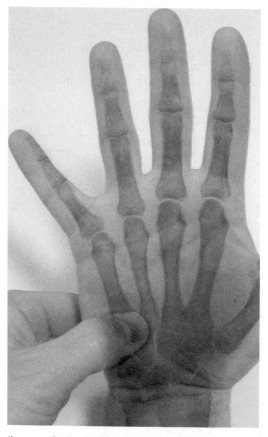

FIG. 3. Direct palpation over the hook of the hamate in the volar palm produces tenderness in cases of hook of the hamate fractures or fracture nonunions.

Radiographic Assessment

Radiographic evaluation of the hook of the hamate can be difficult and requires precise views. The fracture is not seen on a standard AP view because the plane of the fracture is coronal. The fracture may not be appreciated on the lateral view either because of the overlying scaphoid distal pole and trapezium. A 30-degree supinated lateral x-ray may place the hook of the hamate in enough profile so that an unobscured view of the fracture can be seen. A carpal tunnel view may demonstrate the fracture nicely if the patient's pain is not severe. The fracture may be located at the base (most common), midportion, or tip of the hook of the hamate. Often a thin-section spiral CT scan is necessary to make this diagnosis (Fig. 4).

Treatment

Acute or Subacute (<4 Weeks) Fracture

If nondisplaced or minimally displaced, these fractures may be immobilized in an ulnar intrinsic plus cast with the fourth and fifth metaphalangeal (MP) joints in 50 degrees of flexion and the interphalangeal (IP) joints free. Immobilization should continue until 6 weeks after injury. Absence of tenderness and radiographic evidence of early healing should be used as endpoints of immobilization.

Acute Displaced or Chronic Fractures, or Fracture Nonunions

Displaced fractures may be treated with open reduction and internal fixation or with excision of the hook of the hamate. Chronic fractures and fracture

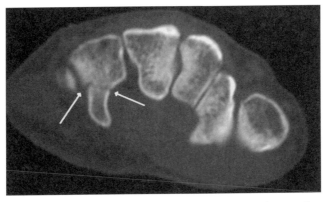

FIG. 4. An axial computed tomography (CT) image demonstrates a fracture *(arrows)* through the base of the hook of the hamate.

nonunions, if symptomatic, are best treated with excision of the hook of the hamate.

Aftercare

Hand therapy is rarely required following closed management of a fracture of the hook of the hamate. Therapy may be beneficial for scar management and strength recovery following open reduction internal fixation (ORIF) or excision of the hook of the hamate.

Key Points

- Patients may have no symptoms with daily activities and pain only when using a club or racket.
- Rarely, a chronic nonunion may be manifested by dysfunction of the small finger secondary to attritional rupture of the flexor pollicis brevis (FDP), which utilizes the radial base of the hook of the hamate as a pulley.

OTHER CARPAL FRACTURES

Diagnostic Criteria

The definitive diagnosis of a carpal bone fracture is made based on positive radiographic and/or other imaging findings. When definitive radiographic evidence of fracture is not present and additional imaging modalities are not available, clinical suspicion should mandate the assumption of fracture until proven otherwise. With a clear history of trauma, other diagnostic considerations include sprains, contusions, dislocations, and ligamentous injuries of the wrist. X-rays and/or additional imaging modalities help distinguish these entities from individual carpal bone fractures.

History

Fractures of the carpal bones are associated with traumatic injuries to the wrist. Although patients with these fractures may present immediately following such an injury, it is not unusual for them to present on a delayed basis. Depending on the nature and severity of the fracture, the patient will complain of pain, swelling, and ecchymosis.

Physical Examination

Depending on the severity of the injury, swelling, ecchymosis, deformity, and limited motion may be present. Localized tenderness is once again a key sign to raise clinical suspicion of a carpal bone fracture. A dorsal triquetral avulsion fracture is a common carpal fracture, the diagnosis of which depends primarily on focal tenderness over the dorsum of the triquetrum. Less common fractures include the trapezium, capitate, lunate, pisiform, trapezoid, and hamate body.

Radiographic Assessment

Standard AP and lateral x-rays are the minimum films required to assess the wrist. Oblique films may be helpful in determining the presence of a subtle fracture that is clinically suspected. A dorsal triquetral avulsion fracture appears as a fleck of bone seen dorsally on the lateral x-ray at the level of the midcarpus. If clinical examination suggests focal tenderness of a single carpal bone and x-rays fail to reveal a fracture, further imaging with a bone scan, CT scan, or MRI may be helpful. If, on plain x-rays, a fracture is noted to extend intraarticularly, a thin-section spiral CT scan with coronal and sagittal reconstructions may be helpful in evaluating the congruity of the articular surface.

Treatment

Nondisplaced carpal fractures generally should be immobilized for a period of approximately 6 weeks. For most fractures, a short-arm cast is appropriate. Trapezium fractures should be immobilized in a thumb spica cast, and consideration should be given to gauntlet cast incorporating the fourth and fifth MP joints for fractures involving the distal portion of the hamate. Triquetral avulsion fractures should be treated similarly to a wrist sprain with a removable cock-up type wrist splint. Progressive mobilization and weaning from a splint should occur following this injury; however, symptoms may persist for 6 weeks or longer. These symptoms tend to decrease over time, but reevaluation is appropriate because stiffness may be a problem and require referral to therapy, or persistent symptoms may be indicative of an additional underlying ligamentous injury.

Displaced fractures may require operative management. The majority of the surface of these carpal bones consists of articular cartilage; therefore, displaced fractures may represent significant articular injuries requiring anatomic reduction. In addition, in a capitate waist fracture, the proximal pole of the capitate may be at increased risk for nonunion because of the retrograde nature of the blood supply to this portion of the capitate. Displaced or nonunited fractures of the pisiform are treated in a similar fashion to hook of the hamate fractures with primary excision rather than ORIF.

Aftercare

Subsequent care, need for therapy, and return to full activities should be dictated by the individual fracture and type of management employed.

Key Points

- Triquetral avulsion fractures may not be seen on the initial lateral x-ray but may be confirmed with a slightly pronated lateral view
- A carpal tunnel view or a slightly supinated lateral x-ray may facilitate the diagnosis of a pisiform fracture.
- The x-rays of a suspected lunate fracture should be inspected carefully for evidence of increased density of the lunate, suggesting that these findings may actually represent fracture or fragmentation of underlying Kienböck's disease.

10

Acute Carpal Dislocations and Ligamentous Injuries

GENERAL INFORMATION

Acute carpal dislocations and acute ligamentous injuries of the wrist represent a spectrum of traumatic injuries to the wrist. Acute carpal dislocations are high-energy injuries to the wrist in which significant ligamentous injury occurs and either radiocarpal or midcarpal dislocation. These injuries may be associated with fracture(s) of the radial styloid, scaphoid, capitate, and/or the triquetrum.

DIAGNOSTIC CRITERIA

Acute Carpal Dislocations

Accurate recognition of the radiographic patterns of acute carpal dislocations leads to prompt diagnosis and elimination of other diagnostic considerations. It is important to recognize acute median nerve compromise when it occurs in the setting of this injury.

Acute Ligamentous Injuries

Early recognition of significant wrist ligament injuries may be difficult because of the subtle nature of radiographic findings. Further evaluation may be appropriate when initial x-rays are normal but clinical examination suggests the possibility of significant ligamentous injury. This may include reevaluation in several days as well as further imaging studies. Magnetic resonance imaging (MRI), arthrography, and MR arthrography may be extremely valuable tools in distinguishing these injuries from severe sprains. The differential diagnosis of acute ligamentous injury to the wrist includes a severe wrist sprain, an occult fracture of the distal radius or a carpal bone, and an acute exacerbation of a chronic ligamentous injury.

History

The mechanism of injury may be varied from severe to relatively minor because these injuries represent a spectrum of injury. Acute carpal dislocations typically are associated with a fall from a height, a motor vehicle accident, or a forceful extension of the wrist by a heavy object. Acute ligamentous injuries may occur by similar mechanisms, as well as by more minor falls and forceful torquing or twisting of the wrist. Acute carpal dislocations produce severe pain and/or visible deformity. Acute ligamentous injuries may produce less immediate pain and no deformity.

Physical Examination

Acute Carpal Dislocations

These injuries usually demonstrate significant deformity, marked soft-tissue swelling, marked limitation in wrist motion secondary to pain, and occasionally, decreased sensation. These injuries are rarely open. Two-point discrimination is diminished in the thumb, index, and long fingers if acute median nerve compromise is present. Carpal canal pressures should not be measured because of possible median nerve displacement.

Acute Ligamentous Injuries

Clinical findings in acute ligamentous injuries may be subtler. Although swelling may be present, it may not be all that impressive. Motion may be decreased secondary to pain during the first several days following injury; however, in the subacute setting, the patient may demonstrate near normal wrist motion but complain of pain at terminal flexion and/or extension. During the acute presentation, tenderness may be diffuse or localized to a specific region of the wrist (e.g., the scapholunate interval). Evaluation of the patient presenting in the subacute setting will more likely reveal focal tenderness. The specific areas to be evaluated for tenderness include the scapholunate interval, the lunotriquetral interval, and the foveal region on the ulnar aspect of the wrist. Specific tests to perform include the Scaphoid Stability test, the lunotriquetral shuck test, the Lichtman maneuver, and assessment of the stability of the distal radial ulnar joint.

Radiographic Assessment

Initial assessment should include standard anterior posterior (AP) and lateral x-rays of the wrist.

Acute Carpal Dislocations

Films should be inspected carefully when these injuries are suspected. Although these dislocations can have several different variations, two primary forms must be recognized. The lateral x-ray is the key to recognizing these patterns. The more easily recognizable pattern is that of a perilunate dislocation. In this situation, the lunate appears to articulate normally or nearly normally with the distal radius, whereas the remaining carpus is dorsally displaced above the lunate and radius (Fig. 1A). In a volar lunate dislocation, the entire carpus appears to have a normal or near normal relationship in regard to the distal radius; however, the lunate is displaced in a volar direction into the carpal canal, and the distal surface is likewise tipped in a volar direction (Figs. 1B and 2). This pattern is easily recognized when compared with a normal lateral x-ray. Associated fractures are usually best recognized on the AP view in acute carpal dislocation. These may include fractures of the radial styloid, scaphoid, capitate, and triquetrum.

Acute Ligamentous Injuries

Radiographic findings in acute ligamentous injuries may be obvious, subtle, or absent. In acute scapholunate ligament injury, attention should be focused on the scapholunate interval on the AP view and the scapholunate angle on the lat-

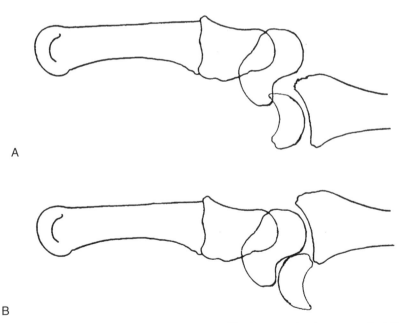

A

B

FIG. 1. A: Lateral view of a perilunate dislocation. The lunate maintains a normal relationship with the distal radius on the lateral view. The remaining carpus is dorsally dislocated about the lunate–radius complex. **B:** Lateral view of a volar lunate dislocation. The carpus dislocates from the lunate and radius and then relocates relative to the radius and forces the lunate to flex in a volar direction and dislocate into the carpal tunnel. This may not be seen clearly on the anterior posterior (AP) view but is well demonstrated on the lateral view.

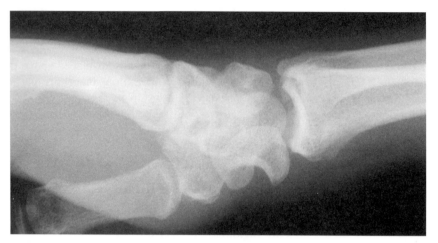

FIG. 2. This lateral x-ray clearly demonstrates that the lunate is displaced and tilted in a volar direction.

eral view. Widening of the scapholunate interval (>4 to 5 mm) is suggestive of acute scapholunate ligamentous injury. Some variation in this interval may be normal, however, and when mild widening is noted, comparison films of the opposite side may be helpful. More subtle widening of this interval may be enhanced by an AP ulnar deviation view of the wrist and/or a "clenched fist" view. The lateral x-ray should be inspected for an increase in the scapholunate angle (Chapter 11, Chronic Carpal Instability). Generally in lunotriquetral, midcarpal, or triangular fibrocartilage complex (TFCC) ligamentous injury, the AP x-rays appear normal. On the lateral view, the carpal malalignment may be noted. Dorsal subluxation of the ulnar head may be seen in significant TFCC ligamentous injury. Note, however, that a slightly oblique lateral view may give a false impression of dorsal prominence of the ulnar head.

TREATMENT

Acute Carpal Dislocations

These injuries require prompt initial treatment. Urgent reduction of the dislocation is necessary to prevent progressive increase in swelling and possible neurovascular compromise. Reduction of a perilunate or lunate dislocation may be attempted in a closed fashion with appropriate sedation. If reduction of the dislocation can be accomplished, definitive treatment of this injury may be delayed for several days; otherwise it should be performed urgently. Definitive treatment should consist of open reduction and internal fixation of fractures, as well as open reduction of the carpal dislocation with pinning of the carpal bones and ligamentous repair.

Acute Ligamentous Injuries

Splinting, ice, and elevation are appropriate before definitive diagnosis is made. Controversy exists regarding treatment of these injuries. The subtler ligamentous injuries (lunotriquetral and midcarpal) may be managed best in a nonoperative fashion. Closed management of acute scapholunate ligamentous injuries generally produces unsatisfactory results. Results following open repair of acute injuries are mixed but usually are more predictable than attempted late reconstruction of chronic injuries.

AFTERCARE

Subsequent care and follow-up of these injuries is dictated by the nature of the definitive treatment provided. A prolonged course of hand therapy and recovery is necessary in almost all cases.

KEY POINTS

- Accurate evaluation of the lateral x-ray is a key element to appropriately diagnosing acute carpal dislocations.
- Appropriate and ongoing assessment of neurovascular status is of paramount importance in the treatment of acute carpal dislocations.
- A high index of suspicion and appropriate further evaluation are necessary to achieve early diagnosis of acute ligamentous injuries.

11

Chronic Carpal Instability

GENERAL INFORMATION

Injuries to the intrinsic and extrinsic carpal ligaments may alter the normal mechanics of the wrist, resulting in pain, disability, and possibly degenerative changes.

DIAGNOSTIC CRITERIA

Establishing the diagnosis of chronic carpal instability may be difficult. Diagnosis is made by synthesis of evaluations from repeated examinations as well as supporting radiographic imaging data.

History

Patients with chronic carpal instability usually present with complaints of pain in the wrist. This may be constant or associated with heavier activities. Their complaints may have been present for weeks, months, or even years. Although some patients may recall a specific injury to their wrist, many are unable to recall any significant injury. Depending on the type of instability (scapholunate, lunotriquetral, midcarpal, etc.), the pain may be located on the radial or ulnar aspect of the wrist. Patients may report a clicking or popping in their wrist with certain activities.

Physical Examination

A detailed examination of the wrist should be performed. This should include objective documentation of range of motion. Pain in certain positions of wrist motion should be noted. Tenderness should be elicited over the first dorsal compartment, the snuffbox, the scapholunate interval, the lunotriquetral interval, the distal radioulnar joint (DRUJ), the triangular fibrocartilage complex (TFCC), the pisotriquetral joint, and the midcarpal joint. Evaluation for

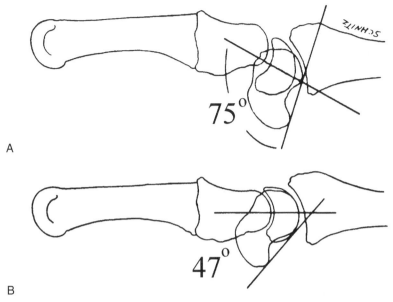

FIG. 1. A: Scapholunate instability is suggested by the increased scapholunate angle. Note the extended position of the lunate. **B:** The normal scapholunate angle is approximately 47 degrees. The lunate is oriented in a neutral tilt position (a line drawn from the peak of its convex surface through the valley of its concave surface is oriented parallel to the long axis of the radius).

instability should be performed with the scapholunate instability, lunotriquetral shuck, and midcarpal instability tests. Comparison with the normal opposite wrist should be made.

Radiographic Assessment

Standard x-rays should include anterior posterior (AP), lateral, and oblique views of the wrist. Additional views for instability include AP ulnar deviation, AP clenched fist, and AP radial deviation. These films should be examined for evidence of carpal instability, fracture, and arthritis. Evidence of scapholunate interval widening and increased scapholunate angle may suggest underlying scapholunate ligament instability (Fig. 1). A mild volar tilt of the lunate may be present with lunotriquetral instability; however, widening of the lunotriquetral interval is uncommon (Fig. 2). These x-rays, in fact, may appear normal in spite of significant underlying instability. Comparison x-rays of the opposite normal wrist may be helpful in evaluating mild changes in carpal alignment (Fig. 3). Frequently, magnetic resonance imaging (MRI), arthrography, and MR arthrography may be required in evaluation of patients with these problems.

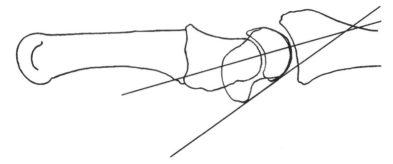

FIG. 2. In lunotriquetral instability the scapholunate angle is decreased and the lunate is in a flexed position (its concave surface is tilted in a volar direction).

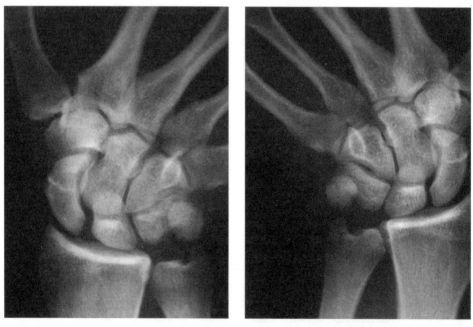

A   B

FIG. 3. A: A slight widening between the scaphoid and lunate on an ulnarly deviated posterior anterior (PA) x-ray suggests scapholunate instability may be present. **B:** Comparison with a similar view of the opposite side demonstrates a normal interval between the scaphoid and lunate.

TREATMENT

Treatment of chronic carpal instability should be tailored to the patient's specific type of instability and degree of symptoms. Significant controversy exists regarding all types of treatment for most types of instability. Although, significant evidence exists to suggest that certain types of chronic instability (scapholunate) are associated with a very high incidence of the late development of post-traumatic arthritis, no conclusive evidence exists to indicate that successful operative reconstruction will prevent such changes from occurring. Nonoperative treatment may be most appropriate for less symptomatic patients. This may include splinting, strengthening, and activity modification. Operative treatment may consist of ligament repair and/or reconstruction, limited arthrodesis, salvage procedures, or complete wrist arthrodesis.

KEY POINTS

- If significant degenerative changes are present radiographically, the patient's condition is longstanding; therefore, his presentation more likely may result from arthritis pain than the underlying instability.
- Patients who have normal ligamentous laxity may develop symptomatic instability from a relatively minor injury.

12

Carpal Metacarpal Fractures and Dislocations

THUMB

Injuries to the carpometacarpal (CMC) region of the thumb include CMC dislocations, simple fracture dislocations (Bennett's fracture), comminuted intraarticular fracture dislocations (Rolando's fracture), and extraarticular fractures of the metacarpal base.

Diagnostic Criteria

Diagnosis is usually not difficult in the case of a Bennett's, Rolando's, or extraarticular fracture of the thumb metacarpal. Radiographic evaluation usually demonstrates conclusively the nature of these injuries.

History

These injuries usually result from a combination of axial loading and an abduction force to the thumb. This may occur during a fall or during a sporting event. A frequent mechanism of injury may be the impact of the thumb against the steering wheel or handlebar during a motor vehicle or cycling accident. If there is more of an axial loading component to the injury, this is more likely to result in a Rolando's-type fracture.

Physical Examination

Evaluation of the thumb and hand generally reveals a substantial amount of swelling in the thenar region. The thumb may appear shortened and/or malrotated. Marked pain in this area may preclude further evaluation; however, crepitance may be noted. It may be possible to feel the CMC joint relocating and resubluxing with manual pressure on the base of the thumb. Accurate diagnosis of the exact nature of the injury is not possible on physical examination alone.

Radiographic Assessment

Anterior posterior (AP) lateral and oblique x-rays of the hand should be obtained. A true lateral of the carpometacarpal (CMC) joint should be obtained as well. A pure CMC dislocation usually represents a dorsal dislocation with disruption of the volar capsular ligaments. A Bennett's fracture demonstrates an intraarticular fracture of the thumb metacarpal base with dorsal subluxation or dislocation of the thumb metacarpal. The size of the volar medial fragment is variable but because of the intact ligamentous structures to this piece, its relationship to the trapezium is usually normal (Fig. 1). A Rolando's fracture is a comminuted fracture on the base of the thumb metacarpal. Typically, this may demonstrate a T- or Y-type pattern, but may be much more comminuted (Fig. 2). The degree of angulation of extraarticular fractures of the thumb metacarpal should be noted on the AP and lateral radiographic views.

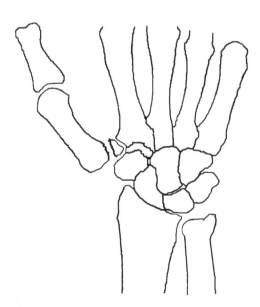

FIG. 1. A Bennett's fracture results in subluxation of the major articular fragment (associates with the metacarpal), whereas the volar medial fragment maintains a normal relationship with the trapezium.

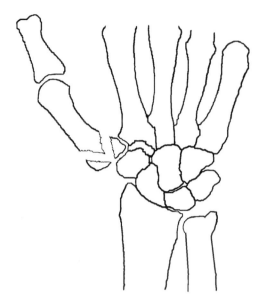

FIG. 2. A Rolando's fracture represents a comminuted intraarticular fracture of the metacarpal base. A Y-type pattern is common.

TREATMENT

Acute treatment of these injuries usually requires appropriate assessment of neurovascular status and temporary immobilization in a thumb spica splint. An attempted reduction should be performed if gross malalignment of the CMC joint is noted. In the case of a pure CMC dislocation, closed reduction is generally possible but significant instability may persist.

A stable CMC reduction and a basilar thumb metacarpal fracture with less than 30 to 40 degrees of angulation and no significant malrotation may both be treated to healing or union in a thumb spica cast. If any question regarding the stability or radiographic assessment of reduction of a CMC dislocation exists, then strong consideration should be given for operative management of this condition. Generally, closed reduction and percutaneous pinning under fluoroscopic guidance is possible. If a basilar metacarpal fracture is malrotated or requires reduction because of significant angulation, then percutaneous pinning or open reduction internal fixation (ORIF) is generally appropriate. Maintenance of a reduction of the thumb metacarpal is difficult with cast treatment alone because of the surrounding soft tissue of the thenar region.

Bennett's and Rolando's fractures require operative management. Frequently, a Bennett's fracture may be managed with closed reduction and percutaneous pinning, especially when the minor fragment is small (Fig. 3). With a larger volar medial fragment, ORIF may be preferable to achieve a more

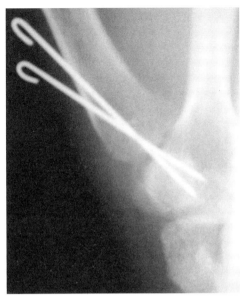

FIG. 3. When the medial fragment is small it is more important to stabilize the major articular fragment relative to the trapezium than to the medial fragment. In this x-ray, anatomic reduction of the carpometacarpal joint has been achieved by pinning the metacarpal base to the trapezium.

anatomic alignment of the articular surface. Treatment of Rolando's fractures can be more challenging and usually requires ORIF and possibly bone grafting. External fixation and percutaneous pinning may be necessary in cases of severe comminution.

AFTERCARE

Aftercare should be tailored to the treatment rendered. Generally, extraarticular fractures in this area heal rapidly, and protected mobilization may begin after 4 weeks. Carpometacarpal dislocations and Bennett's fractures usually require a period of 6 weeks before mobilization. Bennett's and Rolando's fractures treated with ORIF may begin protected mobilization earlier, depending on the assessment of stability at the time of operative treatment.

Late complications of persistent pain and/or the development of arthritis may require additional treatment in the form of CMC arthrodesis or arthroplasty.

KEY POINTS

• The reduction maneuver for the thumb CMC joint is a combination of longitudinal traction, pronation, and dorsal pressure on the thumb metacarpal base.

- In evaluating extraarticular fractures of the thumb metacarpal, one should rely more on clinical evaluation of the thumb in the positions of opposition and abduction than on radiographic criteria alone.
- One should be very critical in evaluating and reevaluating the reduction of a thumb CMC dislocation.

INDEX-SMALL

These injuries involve the metacarpal bases of the index, long, ring, and/or small fingers, with intraarticular involvement. Frequently, a component of CMC subluxation exists, especially in the ring and small rays. Pure CMC dislocation is rare.

Diagnostic Criteria

Clinical suspicion and radiographic evaluation form the foundation for diagnosis of fractures and dislocations of the CMC region. The component of subluxation or dislocation is often missed because of inadequate x-rays and failure to pursue the possibility of such an associated injury. The diagnosis of a fracture in this area is rarely in question. The critical element is determining whether subluxation of the CMC joint is associated with this fracture.

History

Carpometacarpal fractures and dislocations usually occur as a result of an axial load to the hand. A component of hyperextension or hyperflexion of the CMC joint also may be contributory. A common mechanism occurs when a fist strikes a firm or/and immobile object. The patient usually complains of pain, swelling, and limited motion.

Physical Examination

Acute evaluation usually reveals swelling, ecchymosis, and tenderness in the area of injury. If dislocation is associated with this injury, crepitation and/or a sense of relocation/subluxation may be present. Motion is frequently limited secondary to pain. Accurate assessment must be made to evaluate for possible malrotation through the fracture site.

Radiographic Assessment

Standard radiographic views must include AP, lateral, and oblique views of the hand. Radiographic evaluation frequently demonstrates the fracture on an AP view; however, subtle components of subluxation or even dislocation may be difficult to visualize on a lateral x-ray (Fig. 4). A lateral x-ray in slight

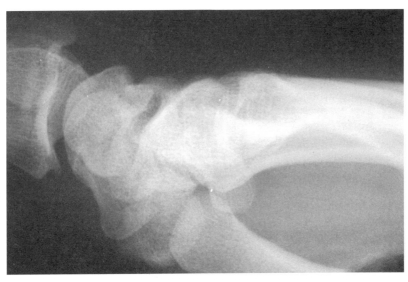

FIG. 4. This x-ray is a lateral of the wrist. It fails to demonstrate any pathology at the small finger carpometacarpal joint.

supination or slight pronation can help isolate and demonstrate the dorsal profile of the index/long and ring/small CMC joints, respectively (Fig. 5). The AP view may be helpful for the assessment of the articular alignment and any degree of step off or subluxation should be noted (Fig. 6). This is particularly difficult for the fourth and fifth CMC joints because of the undulating distal articular surface of the hamate. If any question exists regarding subluxation, dislocation, or significant articular step off, a thin-section spiral computed tomography (CT) scan with coronal and sagittal reconstructions of the CMC joints may be obtained (Fig. 7). CT scan may demonstrate a fracture at either the metacarpal base or the distal articular surface of the carpal bone, especially with regard to the hamate.

TREATMENT

Distinction should be made between fractures of the index and long finger CMC joints and the ring and small finger CMC joints. The index and long finger CMC joints are rigid joints with minimal or no motion; therefore, injury, articular involvement, and minor subluxation may be well tolerated. In contrast, the fourth and fifth CMC joints are highly mobile, and their motion accounts for a large component of the ability of the palm to accommodate to objects of varying size and shape. Residual subluxation or articular step off in these joints is associated with the development of posttraumatic arthrosis.

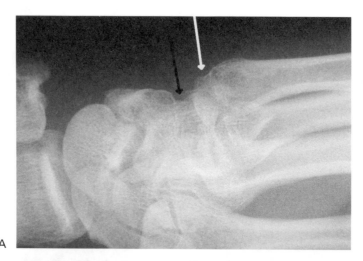

A

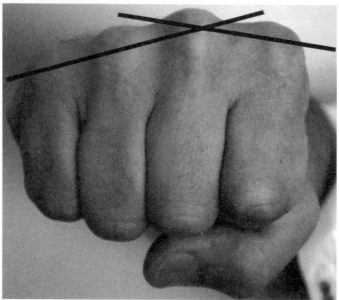

B

FIG. 5. A: A slightly pronated view of the same hand as in Fig. 1 clearly demonstrates the dorsal position of the small finger metacarpal base *(white arrow)* relative to the hamate *(black arrow)*. This represents a dislocation as well as a fracture of the small finger carpometacarpal (CMC) joint. **B:** The index and long finger metacarpals are in a different plane than the ring and small finger metacarpals. A slightly different rotation is required to obtain a true lateral of each pair of CMC joints.

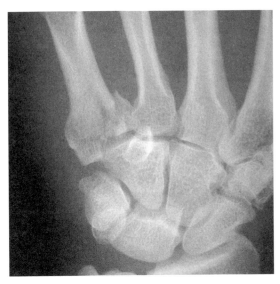

FIG. 6. A fracture dislocation involving the small finger carpometacarpal joint is clearly seen on the AP view.

Nondisplaced intraarticular fractures of any of these CMC joints may be treated with immobilization in an intrinsic plus type cast or splint incorporating the fourth and fifth rays for a period of approximately 4 weeks. If no malrotation is present, mildly to moderately displaced intraarticular fractures and subluxations of the index and long finger CMC joints may be treated in a cast or splint. Late development of pain and/or arthritis following these fractures may be treated with CMC fusion with little or no loss of function.

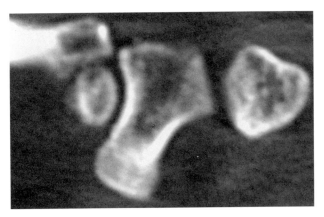

FIG. 7. A sagittal computed tomography image of the small finger carpometacarpal joint demonstrates the fracture and dorsal subluxation of the metacarpal base.

The fourth and fifth CMC joints should be treated more aggressively when significant (>2 mm) articular incongruity, subluxation, or frank dislocation is present. Frequently, this may be managed with closed reduction and percutaneous pinning. Open reduction internal fixation may be necessary if large articular fragments are present and remain significantly displaced following reduction.

KEY POINTS

• One should remember when obtaining and evaluating lateral x-rays, that the index and long finger metacarpals are in one plane and the ring and small finger metacarpals are in a different plane.
• When managing these fractures in a cast or splint or after surgery, the IP joints should be mobilized to avoid stiffness.

13

Fractures and Dislocations of the Metacarpals and Phalanges

GENERAL INFORMATION

Metacarpal and phalangeal fractures are common skeletal injuries that are classified by the pattern of the fracture and the condition of the skin and soft tissues. High-energy injuries cause bone comminution and soft-tissue injury, which adversely affects outcome. This mechanism of injury creates displaced and unstable fractures that often require fracture fixation. In contrast, low-energy injuries cause less damage to the bone and soft-tissue envelope, which makes them more amenable to nonsurgical treatment. The goal of treatment for metacarpal and/or phalangeal fractures is to maintain skeletal length and alignment and restore joint motion.

DIAGNOSTIC CRITERIA

History

A diagnosis of fracture is made by clinical observation confirmed by radiographic findings. The history is important and should include specific details about the amount of force and direction of impact.

Physical Examination

Hand fractures are characterized by pain at the site of fracture, edema, and ecchymoses.

Careful examination of fracture alignment is essential. The finger must be examined both in extension and flexion to detect rotational malalignment. A malrotated finger often appears to be normal in extension, but shows considerable angulation or rotation when examined in flexion (Fig. 1). Comparison

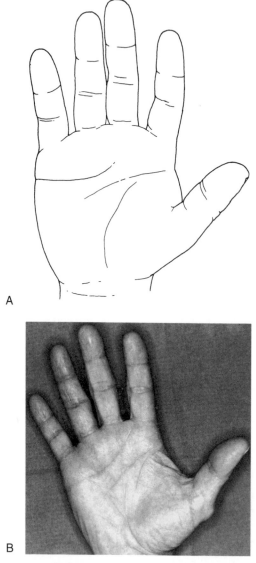

FIG. 1. A: With the finger in extension, a rotational deformity following an index finger proximal phalangeal fracture is not apparent. **B:** Extended right hand of a 50-year-old person with slightly malrotated fracture of the proximal phalanx of the ring finger.

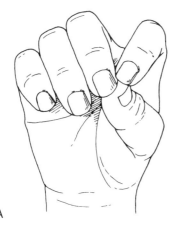

A

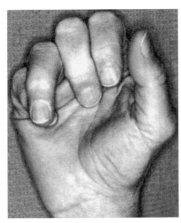

B

FIG. 2. **A:** When the digit is flexed, the deformity is quite apparent. **B:** Active finger flexion generates malrotation of ring finger with digital overlapping.

of the digital cascade between the injured and uninjured hand is also helpful (Fig. 2).

The examination of the fractured extremity should be comprehensive. A notation about the soft tissues is necessary, including the ligamentous stability, tendon integrity, skin condition, vascular supply, and neurologic condition.

Radiographic Assessment

Anteroposterior and lateral x-rays are required to determine the pattern of fracture. The injury site should be centered on the radiographic cassette. Lateral x-rays of the digits can be difficult to obtain. To acquire a more accurate lateral view of the injured finger, one should raise it away from the rest of the digits or rotate the hand. Advanced imaging modalities (e.g., computed tomography [CT] or magnetic resonance imaging [MRI]) are not necessary for initial fracture evaluation.

TABLE 1. *Clear descriptors for metacarpal and phalangeal fractures*

Nondisplaced	Displaced
Stable	Unstable
Reducible	Irreducible
Extraarticular	Intraarticular
Simple	Comminuted
Closed	Open

COMMUNICATING ABOUT FRACTURES

When discussing fractures with colleagues, one should use unambiguous terms with precise meaning. Describing fractures by using traditional fracture classification systems and fracture eponyms has significant problems. Fracture classification systems often are associated with significant rates of interobserver error, do not direct treatment, and are not predictive of outcome. Rather than using fracture eponyms and classification systems, it is better to use basic terms that clearly describe the injury. First, one should describe the location of the injury by identifying the fractured bone and the location of the injury within the bone (intraarticular or extraarticular). Second, one should define the fracture as simple (single fracture line) or comminuted (multiple fracture lines). Third, one should determine whether the fracture is displaced or not displaced and measure the amount of displacement and angulation between the two fracture ends (Table 1). Finally, one must communicate the status of the soft-tissue injury or other circumstance that may affect the treatment pathway.

DETERMINATION OF FRACTURE HEALING

Fracture healing is determined by clinical and radiographic criteria. A fracture site that is nontender is healed enough to allow active digital range of motion. Most fractures treated by nonoperative methods heal by the formation of callus at the fracture site (secondary bone healing). An early radiographic sign of union is fracture "callus" that bridges the bone ends. Later the callus will organize and "bridging trabeculae" of more mature bone will be seen crossing the site of fracture. Fractures that are treated with rigid plate fixation may undergo a different kind of bone healing (primary bone union) that heals with very little or no callus formation. In general, radiographic findings lag well behind clinical findings.

NONDISPLACED FRACTURES OR STABLE INJURIES

Stable, nondisplaced, closed metacarpal and phalangeal fractures are immobilized in a functional position for 10 to 14 days. The patient is then begun on a

TABLE 2. *General fracture care*

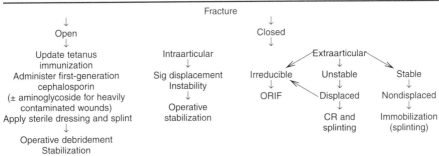

CR, closed reduction; ORIF, open reduction internal fixation.

program to restore active range of motion (Tables 2 and 3). Hand immobilization must resist the muscular forces that may cause the fracture to displace and place the joints in their "best" position. The intrinsic muscles are the primary deforming forces in most metacarpal and proximal phalanx fractures. These muscles bend the fractured metacarpal into an apex dorsal angulation and the fractured proximal phalanx into an apex volar angulation (Fig. 3). To keep the ligamentous structures of the metacarpophalangeal (MCP) joint at their maximum length, these joints should be immobilized in 50 to 70 degrees of flexion

TABLE 3. *General principles of initial fracture management*

Careful assessment
  History
  Physical examination
  Skeletal examination
    Tenderness
    Ecchymoses
    Digit alignment
    Stability testing
  Skin examination
  Vascular examination
  Neurologic examination
  Tendon examination
  Radiographs
Immobilization
Ice
Elevation of the limb
Pain management
  Nonsteroidal antiinflammatory medication drug
  Analgesic medication
Instructions for home care
Contact person for interim problems
Coordination of follow-up for definitive care
  Open fractures need immediate assessment
  Most closed fractures should be evaluated 3 to 7 days following injury

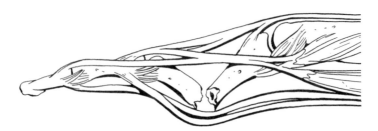

FIG. 3. The intrinsic muscle causes flexion deformity of phalanx fracture.

(otherwise, they are prone to develop an extension contracture). In contrast, the interphalangeal joints are prone to develop flexion contractures. To keep the ligaments of the interphalangeal joints stretched to their maximum length, these joints should be positioned in extension. Fortunately, this position of MCP flexion and interphalangeal joint extension (i.e., the intrinsic plus position) both relaxes the intrinsic muscles and places the joints in a desirable position.

DISPLACED FRACTURES

A displaced metacarpal or phalangeal fracture that is able to be reduced and is stable following reduction is usually treated by application of an appropriately positioned splint. Following reduction, the digit should be examined in flexion and extension to ensure that an accurate reduction has been obtained. Criteria visible on plain radiographs for an acceptable reduction are the following: less than 10 degrees of coronal angulation, less than 5 mm of shortening, and at least 50% of accurate cortical apposition at the fracture site. Acceptable sagittal plane deformity depends on the finger involved. More angulation is tolerable in the ring and small digits because of greater carpometacarpal joint motion compared with the index and long fingers. In general, sagittal angulation of 30 degrees more than the available carpometacarpal motion is acceptable. Successful closed reduction is followed by immobilization in the intrinsic plus position for 3 to 4 weeks. Buddy taping can then be used both to control rotation and promote return of motion. Closed reduction and splinting can usually be done in the emergency department using nerve block and/or intravenous sedation.

DISPLACED AND UNSTABLE FRACTURES

A displaced metacarpal or phalangeal fracture with an unstable fracture configuration is usually treated by closed reduction and stabilization of the bone, using percutaneously placed wires or screws (Fig. 4). The initial treatment is the same as for displaced fractures with an attempt at closed reduction. The tech-

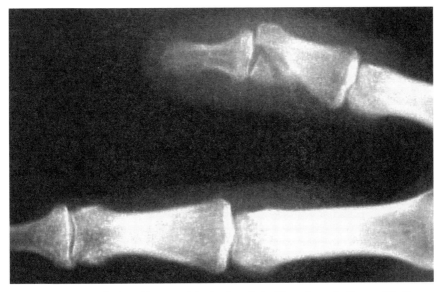

FIG. 4. Unstable displaced intercondylar fracture that will require reduction and fixation.

nique of open reduction and internal fixation is another treatment consideration for displaced and unstable metacarpal and phalangeal fractures. Definitive open reduction and fracture fixation is best done between 7 and 10 days following injury to allow for a reduction in swelling and is usually performed in an operating room.

FRACTURES THAT CANNOT BE REDUCED USING CLOSED METHODS

A displaced, irreducible metacarpal or phalangeal fracture requires an open reduction and internal fixation of the fracture fragments. Accurate fracture alignment is established by direct inspection, and is subsequently stabilized with wires and screws or plates and screws. Most irreducible fractures (especially those with significant soft-tissue injuries) need urgent treatment.

OPEN FRACTURES

To limit the risk for infection, open fractures must be thoroughly irrigated and the bone ends débrided. Open fractures can be further subdivided by the size of the wound, level of contamination, and presence or absence of a vascular injury. Patients with these types of fractures require emergency evaluation and treatment. Typically these fractures require external or internal fixation.

INTRAARTICULAR FRACTURES

Metacarpophalangeal Joint

Intraarticular fractures of the MCP joint are uncommon. The extent of articular involvement and degree of joint instability are the parameters that guide treatment. Mild joint incongruity (i.e., 1 mm or less) can be accepted as long as joint stability is preserved. Greater degrees of joint step-off or joint instability require open reduction and internal fixation.

Proximal Interphalangeal Joint

Intraarticular fractures of the proximal interphalangeal (PIP) joint are commonly associated with dorsal subluxation or dislocation (Fig. 5). Small avulsion fractures from the palmar base of the middle phalanx (often called volar plate avulsion injuries) are treated similar to a PIP joint dislocation. Immobilization for a few days followed by early motion optimizes outcome. Prolonged immobilization should be avoided to minimize stiffness and a PIP joint contracture. Larger fractures of the middle phalanx palmar base (25% to 30%) can disrupt the collateral ligament insertions and are associated with dorsal subluxation during extension (Fig. 5). Closed reduction and extension block splinting allows early motion and prevents subluxation of the joint. The technique for extension block splinting requires a short-arm cast and a dorsal outrigger (aluminum-foam splint), which is incorporated into the cast (Fig. 6). The outrigger extends over the injured digit and places the MCP joint in 70 to 80 degrees of flexion and the PIP joint in enough flexion to achieve concentric joint reduction. Lateral x-rays taken after cast application that are centered on the proximal interphalangeal joint establish that the PIP joint reduction is accurate. Active finger flexion and extension is encouraged within the cast to the limit of the extension block. Over

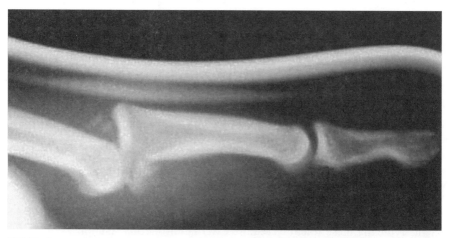

FIG. 5. An unreduced proximal interphalangeal fracture dislocation that will require closed or open reduction.

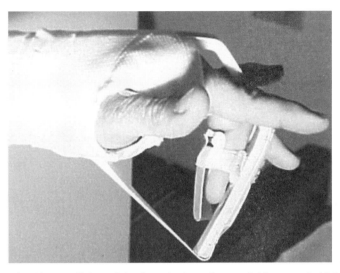

FIG. 6. Dorsal outrigger splint consists of an aluminum-foam splint incorporated into a cast. In the section of the aluminum splint that is incorporated in the cast, the foam should be removed.

the next 4 to 5 weeks, the dorsal outrigger is adjusted weekly to allow increasing amounts of extension (10 to 15 degrees per week). After each splint adjustment, another lateral x-ray is taken to confirm reduction of the proximal interphalangeal joint. Fracture fragments that are more than 30% of the joint surface of the middle phalanx may not be amenable to extension block splinting and may require operative treatment. Residual loss of motion and joint degeneration are common in comminuted intraarticular fractures that involve more than 30% of the joint.

Distal Interphalangeal Joint

Intraarticular fractures of the distal phalanx are associated with avulsion injuries of the flexor or extensor tendons. A palmar avulsion fracture signifies a flexor tendon avulsion and requires early surgery for tendon reattachment. A dorsal avulsion fracture (bony mallet fracture) (Fig. 7) is treated by splint appli-

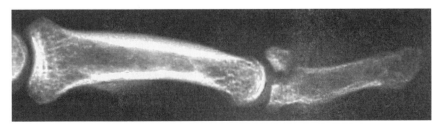

FIG. 7. Bony mallet fracture that can be treated in a splint.

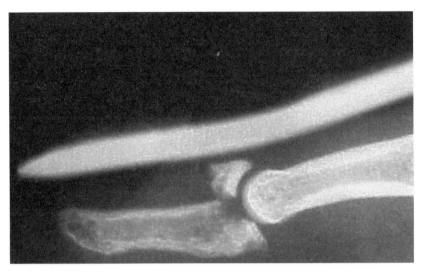

FIG. 8. Bony mallet fracture with joint subluxation that will require reduction and stabilization.

cation. The DIP joint is held in extension for 6 to 8 weeks. Surgical treatment for a bony mallet injury is usually reserved for those that involve palmar subluxation of the DIP joint (Fig. 8). Injuries that have a large dorsal fragment that includes a considerable amount of the articular surface may also require open reduction and internal fixation.

JOINT DISLOCATIONS

Metacarpophalangeal Joint

Metacarpophalangeal joint dislocations are relatively rare. When they do occur, they most commonly involve the thumb, index, and long fingers. The proximal phalanx is usually displaced in a dorsal direction. "Complex" dislocations are those that cannot be reduced by closed manipulation (Fig. 9). In complex dislocations of the index and long fingers, the palmar plate is often interposed in the joint, and the metacarpal head is trapped between the flexor tendons and the lumbrical muscle. Open reduction is required to restore alignment and joint congruity. Immobilization for 1 to 2 weeks following surgery is usually necessary to restore stability.

Proximal Interphalangeal Joint

Proximal interphalangeal joint dislocations are common. The middle phalanx usually dislocates in a dorsal direction (Table 4). Reduction is performed under

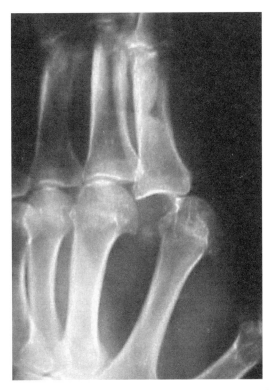

FIG. 9. Complex metaphalangeal dislocation that was unable to be reduced by closed means.

digital block by using longitudinal traction. Following reduction, the PIP joint is usually stable throughout the full range of motion. X-rays following reduction should be taken to ensure that a concentric reduction has been obtained. A short period of immobilization (3 to 10 days) in slight flexion or immediate active motion is appropriate. Recurrent dorsal dislocation on extension requires exten-

TABLE 4. *Proximal interphalangeal joint dislocations*

Dislocation[a]	Reduction	Splint
Dorsal	Axial traction and flexion of the distal fragment	10 degrees of flexion
Lateral	Axial traction and lateral or medial repositioning of the joint	10 degrees of flexion
Volar	Wrist in extension, MCP and PIP joints in flexion. Longitudinal traction applied to the distal fragment and lifted into a reduced position	Full extension
Volar rotational	May be irreducible secondary to soft tissue interposition	Depends on method of operative stabilization

[a]The direction of dislocation is commonly defined by the position of the most distal bone. For example, if the middle phalanx is dorsally displaced, then it is referred to as a dorsal dislocation. *MCP*, metacarpophalangeal; *PIP*, proximal interphalangeal.

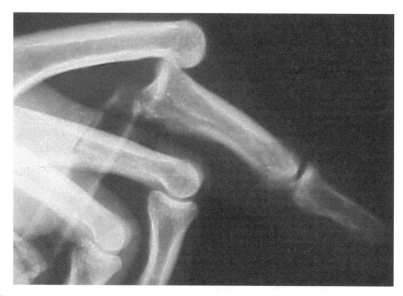

FIG. 10. A palmar dislocation of the proximal interphalangeal (PIP) joint that can be treated with closed reduction and splinting. The PIP joint is maintained in extension for 6 weeks to allow the central slip to heal.

sion block splinting, similar to that for a PIP joint fracture. Palmar dislocation of the middle phalanx is less common and is associated with an injury to the central slip of the extensor tendon (Fig. 10). Treatment is joint reduction and splinting for 5 to 6 weeks in extension to allow healing of the central slip.

Distal Interphalangeal Joint

Distal interphalangeal joint dislocations are rare. The distal phalanx usually displaces in a dorsal direction. Preferred treatment is closed reduction using longitudinal traction. Postreduction x-rays should be taken to ensure that a concentric reduction has been obtained.

OTHER SPECIFIC INJURIES

Boxer's Fracture

A "Boxer's fracture" is a fracture of the distal metaphysis of the ring or small finger metacarpal, which has an apex dorsal angulation (Fig. 11). Examination shows tenderness over the fracture site and loss of the normal metacarpal head prominence. Because of the mobility of the carpometacarpal joint, considerable sagittal plane angulation (up to 60 degrees) is acceptable in the small digit. Closed reduction is usually performed for a fracture that is angulated more than 30 degrees to restore metacarpal head contour. The fracture is immobilized in a

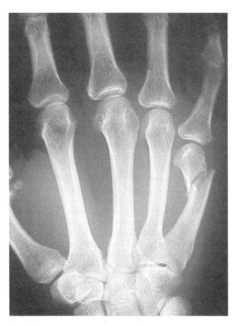

FIG. 11. A "Boxer's fracture" that can be treated with closed reduction and splinting for approximately 4 weeks.

forearm-based ulnar gutter cast or splint that positions the ring and small digits in the intrinsic plus position for 4 to 6 weeks. Surgery is rarely necessary for this fracture. The carpometacarpal joints of the index and long are less mobile, and angular deformities of metacarpal neck fractures are not as well tolerated. A more precise reduction is required to prevent residual displacement at the fracture site. Failure to correct the malalignment causes a prominent metacarpal head in the palm, which interferes with gripping activities. Closed reduction of displaced index and long finger metacarpal neck fractures is recommended to restore metacarpal alignment.

Fractures of the Base of the Little Finger Metacarpal

Because of the pull of the extensor carpi ulnaris, fractures involving the base of the little finger metacarpal are often unstable and require operative stabilization. After initial immobilization in an ulnar gutter splint, these fractures should be referred for urgent reevaluation.

Gamekeeper's or Skier's Thumb

A tear of the ulnar collateral ligament of the thumb is referred to as a gamekeeper's or skier's thumb. A valgus stress applied to the thumb MCP joint disrupts the ligament, usually from the proximal phalanx (Fig. 12). Partial ligament injuries are usually stable when stressed into valgus. The intact fibers of the ulnar collateral ligament provide an endpoint to a valgus stress. Partial collateral ligament injuries are treated by immobilization for 2 to 3 weeks. A completely torn ligament completely disrupts the integrity of the ulnar collateral ligament. Patients with complete ligament tears are unstable (i.e., possess no endpoint when stress is applied to the ulnar collateral ligament of the MCP) when tested in full MCP extension and 30 degrees of MP flexion. This torn ligament may displace outside the adductor aponeurosis (a.k.a. Stener's lesion) and is not able to heal properly (Fig. 13). The Stener lesion may be palpable near the ulnar side of the metacarpal head as a mass, which is the retracted ligament. Complete tears require surgical exploration to evaluate the position of the ligament and reattach the ligament to the proximal phalanx. When possible, the surgery should be performed within 10 days of injury. Chronic complete tears are associated with per-

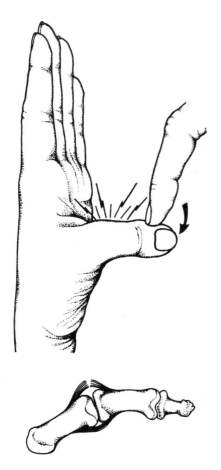

FIG. 12. Rupture of ulnar collateral ligament of the metacarpophalangeal joint of the thumb.

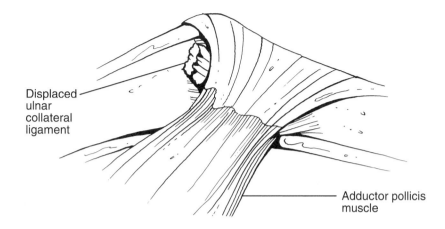

Displaced ulnar collateral ligament

Adductor pollicis muscle

FIG. 13. Stener's lesion occurs when the ulnar collateral ligament is displaced proximal to the adductor aponeurosis. When the ruptured ligament is in this position, chronic metacarpophalangeal joint instability can occur.

sistent pain, instability, and early arthritis. Ligament reconstruction can be performed prior to joint degeneration, although results are inferior to those obtained after immediate repair. Metacarpophalangeal joint arthritis in the presence of instability requires arthrodesis to ameliorate the symptoms.

KEY POINTS

- The goal of fracture treatment is to obtain a stable reduction of the bone that allows range of motion to occur within a reasonable amount of time.
- Most closed stable fractures should be reassessed within 7 to 10 days following injury to ensure no displacement.
- Urgent reevaluation (1 to 2 days) should be recommended to patients who have injuries that may need operative treatment.
- Open fractures, fractures with significant soft-tissue injury (i.e., compartment syndrome), and irreducible injuries require emergency treatment.

SELECTED REFERENCES

Dabezies EJ, Schutte JP. Fixation of metacarpal and phalangeal fractures with miniature plates and screws. J Hand Surg 1986;11A:283–288.
Green DP, Anderson JR. Closed reduction and percutaneous pin fixation of fractured phalanges. J Bone Joint Surg 1973;55A:1651–1654.
Kozin SH, Thoder JJ, Lieberman G. Operative treatment of metacarpal and phalangeal shaft fractures. J Am Acad Orthop Surg 2000;8:111–121.
Stern PJ. Management of fractures of the hand over the last 25 years. J Hand Surg 2000;25A:817–823.
Wehbe MA, Schneider LH. Mallet fractures. J Bone Joint Surg Am 1984;66:658–669.

14

Soft-Tissue Injuries and Lacerations

GENERAL INFORMATION

Soft-tissue wounds to the hand are common. These injuries vary from simple, clean, sharp superficial lacerations to deep, severely contaminated crush injuries. Use of the terms lacerations or open wounds implies that the skin barrier has been violated. Bacterial contamination, with superficial and deep soft-tissue damage, may have occurred. Optimal treatment of these injuries requires obtaining an adequate history along with a systematic physical evaluation of the extremity. The history should include general information concerning the patient (e.g., age, hand dominance, comorbid medical conditions, tetanus status) in addition to information about the injury itself. Socioeconomic factors (e.g., work injuries, self-inflicted injuries) may also play a role in the treatment of these injuries.

The initial treatment of these injuries should include using sterile, compressive dressings and elevation of the hand to control bleeding if present. The use of hemostats, placed into the wound to control bleeding, should be avoided. A careful assessment of the entire extremity and not only the injured area should be performed.

DIAGNOSTIC CRITERIA

History

The history should include the anatomic location of the injury, time since injury, the mechanism of injury, where the injury occurred (e.g., kitchen versus field), presence of numbness or paresthesias, presence of any bleeding from the wound, and any previous injuries or treatment.

Physical Examination

An adequate assessment of a hand laceration should include an inspection of the hand. That assessment would include noting the resting hand posture (e.g., presence or absence of a normal hand cascade), any skin discoloration, presence of swelling, erythema, bleeding; and the location of the wound (e.g., dorsal or volar).

The physical examination should include an examination of joint motion (active and passive), status of the flexor and extensor tendons, motor and sensory (two-point sensory examination of all digits) examination, and vascular examination (palpation of pulses, Allen's test). An examination is critical prior to the use of any local or regional anesthetics.

The location and depth of the wound(s) then should be assessed. Local anesthetics using plain lidocaine (without epinephrine) may be needed to adequately assess the wounds. Adequate equipment (tourniquet, surgical instruments, lighting) is needed to fully assess a deep wound.

X-rays of any area of injury, particularly those with open wounds, should be performed to visualize foreign bodies or osseous injuries.

TREATMENT

In general, wounds that are over 6 hours old should not be closed. Open treatment or healing by secondary intention is very useful for infected hand wounds and chronic open wounds (Table 1). Simple, clean wounds may be débrided, irrigated, and closed. Heavily contaminated wounds also should be débrided, irrigated, packed, and left open. Débridement of damaged and contaminated tissues is important in proper wound management. Irrigation of the wound should be performed using a pulsating jet lavage irrigation system.

Antibiotic coverage may not be needed in the treatment of simple, clean wounds. Wounds with a higher risk of infection (e.g., human or animal bites, penetrating wounds, crush wounds, or contaminated wounds) should have antibiotic coverage. These wounds should also have aerobic and anaerobic cultures taken at the time of débridement. In general, a first-generation cephalosporin (e.g., Ancef, Kefzol) or penicillinase-resistant penicillin (e.g., Nafcillin, Oxacillin, Methicillin) can be used (Table 2).

The most common pathogens for human bites include *Staphylococcus aureus, Streptococcus, Eikenella corrodens,* and *Bacteroides B.* Antibiotic coverage includes Penicillin G and Cefazolin, Timentin, Unasyn, or Augmentin (Amoxicillin plus K-clavulanate). Animal bites should be covered for *Pasturella multo-*

TABLE 1. *Open treatment for hand wounds*

Frequency: two to three times a day
Use sterile methods
Clean wound with solution of normal saline (three parts) and hydrogen peroxide (one part)
  (Add a small amount of Betadine if the wound is dirty.)
Rinse the wound and then cover (or pack) with saline-soaked gauze
Apply top dressing and splint
Reevaluate wound frequently

TABLE 2. *Cephalosporins*

First generation	Second generation	Third generation
Cephalothin (Keflin, Seffin)	Cefamandole (Mandole)	Cefotaxime (Claforan)
Cephapirin (Cefadyl)	Cefoxitin (Mefoxin)	Ceftizoxime (Cefizox)
Cephradine (Anspor, Velosef)	Cefuroxime (Zinacef, Kefurox)	Ceftriaxone (Rocephin)
Cefazolin (Ancef, Kefzol)	Cefonicid (Monocid)	Cefmenoxime (Cefmax)
For oral use	Cefotetan (Cefotan)	Moxalactam (Moxam)
Cephalexin (Keflex)	Ceforanide (Precef)	Cefoperazone (Cefobid)
Cephradine (Anspor, Velosef)		Ceftazidime (Fortaz,
Cefadroxil (Duncef, Ultracef)		Tazidime, Tazicef)
Cefaclor (Ceclor)		Cefsulodin (Cefomonid)

cida in addition to *S. aureus* and *Streptococcus,* and should have antibiotic coverage similar to human bites.

Heavily contaminated wounds may require the additional use of an aminoglycoside (e.g., Gentamicin, Tobramycin, Amikacin) or a second- or third-generation cephalosporin (e.g., Clindamycin, Vancomycin).

Tetanus prophylaxis should be used for most open hand wounds. In general, those patients who have not been previously immunized; have not had a booster injection within the past 5 years; or have a contaminated wound, need a tetanus toxoid booster, tetanus immune globulin, or both (Table 3).

PUNCTURE WOUNDS

Puncture wounds can be caused by a variety of materials (e.g., metal, glass, wood, teeth). Knowledge of the exact mechanism of injury is critical. Wounds associated with minimal contamination (e.g., glass) can be treated with local wound irrigation and débridement of necrotic skin edges. Formal surgical exploration in an appropriate environment should be performed if a foreign body is suspected but is not directly visible within the wound margins. Wounds that are associated with a potentially high degree of contamination (e.g., human bites)

TABLE 3. *Tetanus immunization schedule recommended by the US Public Health Service*

Tetanus immunization history (doses)	Clean minor wounds, toxoid	Clean minor wounds, TIG	All other wounds, toxoid	All other wounds, TIG
Uncertain	Yes	No	Yes	Yes
0–1	Yes	No	Yes	Yes
2	Yes	No	Yes	No[a]
3	No[b]	No	No[c]	No

[a]Unless wound is more than 24 hours old.
[b]Unless more than 10 years since last toxoid dose.
[c]Unless more than 5 years since last toxoid dose.
TIG, Tetanus immune globulin (human); *toxoid,* tetanus toxoid.

should undergo formal surgical exploration and débridement. With injuries overlying joints, the surgical exploration should ensure that joint penetration has not occurred. An arthrotomy and joint irrigation should be performed if the injury has entered the joint.

High-pressure injection injuries (e.g., paints, lubricants, abrasives, solvents) require open débridement of the area of injury (Chapter 27, High-Pressure Injection Injuries). Repeat débridements frequently are required.

Gunshot wounds secondary to low-velocity missiles (e.g., .22-caliber weapon), usually can be treated with local wound care and a careful assessment of injuries to underlying structures. Wounds secondary to high-energy missiles (e.g., rifles, close-range shotgun injuries) or those missiles moving more than 2,000 ft/second need formal exploration, débridement, and irrigation. These injuries are frequently associated with significant soft-tissue and skeletal injuries requiring later reconstructive work.

VOLAR AND DORSAL HAND WOUNDS

Injuries to the flexor tendons and neurovascular structures should be suspected with volar hand wounds. Deep wounds, in addition to a careful preoperative assessment, require thorough débridement and irrigation of the wound and careful inspection and repair of injured structures.

Extensor tendon lacerations should be suspected with dorsal wounds. Human bite lacerations should be considered with injuries over the metacarpophalangeal joint. Joint contamination may be present in addition to extensor mechanism injuries.

CRUSH, BURST, AVULSION, AND DEGLOVING WOUNDS

When compared with simple wounds, these complex injuries are associated with a higher degree of soft-tissue injury, which results in more edema, fibrosis, and stiffness. The basics of treatment include débridement and irrigation, skeletal stabilization, soft-tissue reconstruction, skin coverage, and early mobilization.

KEY POINTS

- Careful wound assessment is essential to treatment.
- Open treatment is very useful for hand wounds that are infected or have been open for more than 6 hours. In general, wounds that are infected require more frequent dressing changes. These wounds also may need wound irrigation with bacteriocidal agents such as Betadine when they are dirty or infected. Clean wounds may need lavage only with normal saline and saline gauze dressings.

For further information see Chapter 27 (High-Pressure Injection Injuries) and 28 (Bites).

15

Extensor Tendon Injuries

GENERAL INFORMATION

Tendon Laceration

The extensor tendons are divided into eight zones (Fig. 1). Odd-numbered zones are on the joints and even zones are between the joints. Zone 1 is over the distal interphalangeal (DIP) joint.

The extensor mechanism is a finely balanced system that requires two muscles to extend three joints. Elongation or shortening over the digit as little as 3 mm may produce significant changes in the range of motion.

Partial Tendon Laceration

Tendon lacerations of less than 50% of the diameter of the tendon are usually asymptomatic and do not need repair; however, when a partial laceration occurs at the central slip insertion, failure to repair it will lead to palmar subluxation of the lateral bands (boutonniere).

Mallet Finger

A mallet finger is loss of active extension of the DIP joint. There are three causes of a mallet finger: tendon transection distal to the proximal interphalangeal (PIP) joint, tendon avulsion from the distal phalanx, and fracture of the distal phalanx with associated loss of extensor insertion site. With proximal retraction of the extensor apparatus, there can be associated PIP joint extension (swan neck deformity).

Boutonniere Injury

A boutonniere deformity is loss of active extension of the PIP joint with subsequent hyperextension of the DIP joint. There are three causes of a boutonniere deformity in the finger: tendon transection between the metaphalangeal (MP) and PIP joints, tendon avulsion from its insertion into the base of the middle pha-

118

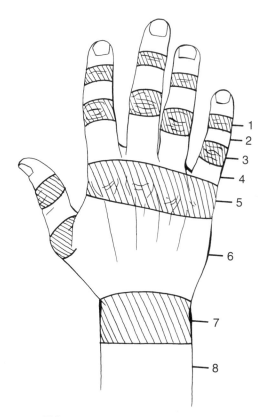

FIG. 1. Zones of extensor tendon injury.

lanx, and fracture of the dorsal lip of the middle phalanx with associated loss of extensor continuity. When a boutonniere injury occurs, the extensor apparatus retracts proximally and the lateral bands translate to a position that is now below the axis of PIP joint rotation, making them flexors of the PIP joint. As they move in a palmar direction, they also cause increased tension on the DIP joint, which increases resting extension in the DIP joint.

DIAGNOSTIC CRITERIA

Laceration of the extensor surface of the wrist, hand, and forearm can be complicated by tendon transection because the extensor mechanism is very close to the skin on the dorsum of the hand. The extensor tendon can also be ruptured by forcibly flexing a digit that is trying to extend (closed mallet injury, closed boutonniere injury). Establish the status of tetanus immunization if a laceration has been sustained.

First inspect the hand for abnormal posturing of the digit. Specifically, inspect the hand for loss of DIP, PIP, and metacarpophalangeal (MCP) joint extension.

Next, check passive motion of the joints with wrist in extension and flexion (tenodesis, effect, anatomy, and physical examination). Finally, assess active digital extension of the MCP, PIP, and DIP joints. Inability to extend the joint is consistent with complete tendon transection. Painful digital extension is consistent with partial tendon transection. Carefully document the position and depth of the laceration and consider the possibility of an associated injury to the joint capsule.

OTHER ASSESSMENT(S)

Plain radiographs are helpful, especially in cases without a laceration (closed mallet and closed boutonniere) to determine if a significant bony avulsion has occurred. Uncommonly, patients with terminal extensor tendon rupture (mallet finger) will have a dislocation or subluxation of the DIP joint. Patients with significant dorsal articular fractures of the middle phalanx at the PIP joint will commonly have joint subluxation.

TREATMENT

Laceration and Tendon Injury

Initial Treatment

As with any wound, the patient's tetanus immunization status should be updated. The wound should be irrigated and débrided and the deep tissues inspected to determine the status of the extensor tendon. The digit should be carefully flexed and extended to determine whether the joint is open. If both tendon ends are visualized, the laceration may be repaired. If the surgeon is unable to repair the tendon, the wound is closed and the hand and fingers are splinted in extension.

Definitive Treatment

Tendon repair of the digit often can be performed in the emergency room setting using a digital anesthetic and tourniquet. The tendon should be repaired within 7 to 10 days if delayed primary repair is chosen. Proximal and distal wound extensions allow identification of the tendon ends. The tendon is repaired after mobilization. Extensor tendons are commonly repaired using a 4-0 or 3-0 braided Dacron or monofilament suture. In zones 1 to 4, the tendon is repaired with a figure of eight or mattress suture. In zones 5 to 8, a two-strand suture method (modified Kessler method) is used (Fig. 2).

Tendon retraction may occur in injuries proximal to the juncturae or in the extensor pollicis longus (EPL). The proximal tendon may retract to beneath the wrist retinaculum. The repair should be done in the operating room when tendon

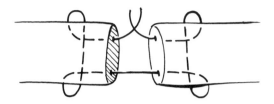

FIG. 2. Two-strand tendon repair (modified Kessler method).

retrieval is difficult, the wound is complicated, or there are significant associated injuries.

The zone of injury determines the type of postoperative dressing. In general, the DIP is immobilized in zone 1 and 2 injuries, and the PIP and DIP are immobilized in zone 3 and 4 injuries. In zone 5 to 8 injuries, the MP joints are immobilized in full extension and the wrist in 10 degrees of extension.

Closed Tendon Avulsion Injuries

Mallet

Treatment is continuous extension splinting of the distal interphalangeal joint for 6 weeks. If there is a bony injury, x-rays should be done to ensure concentric joint reduction of the distal interphalangeal joint. If significant joint subluxation develops or if the articular fragment is greater than 40% of the joint surface (on the lateral x-ray), then operative treatment should be considered.

Boutonniere

The PIP joint should be splinted in continuous extension for 6 weeks if treatment is instituted early. Treatment options include prolonged splinting and/or surgery for patients who present for evaluation with a chronic injury.

AFTERCARE

Tendon Repair

There are a number of protocols for aftercare following extensor tendon repair. The affected region is splinted for 3 to 4 weeks, after which range of motion exercises are initiated. Intensive occupational therapy may be necessary for 6 to 12 weeks.

A tenolysis and joint release may be considered at 3 to 6 months following treatment if there is significant stiffness following successful tendon repair.

KEY POINTS

- Patients with a dorsal hand laceration and inability to extend a joint should be presumed to have a tendon transection.
- Patients with a dorsal hand laceration and painful motion should have the wound explored prior to closure looking for a tendon laceration.
- Patients with a closed flexion injury of a joint who have inability to extend the DIP or PIP should be presumed to have an extensor apparatus avulsion (mallet or boutonniere).

SELECTED REFERENCE

Newport ML, Blair WF, Steyers CM. Long-term results of extensor tendon repair. J Hand Surg 1990; 15A:961–966.

16

Flexor Tendon Injuries

GENERAL INFORMATION

Lacerations to the palmar surface of the digit and hand are frequently complicated by injury to the flexor tendons. In general, tendon injuries are classified as partial lacerations, complete lacerations, and tendon avulsion injuries.

DIAGNOSTIC CRITERIA

History

Most patients present for evaluation of a laceration to the palmar surface of the hand that is associated with a loss of active digital flexion. Some patients with partial tendon injury may describe painful digital flexion. Depending on the location of the laceration there may be associated loss of digital sensibility and loss of motor strength. Inquire about tetanus immunization and other drug sensitivities should be determined. The position of the hand at the time of the injury (i.e., gripping a knife) may give some insight into the position of the distal tendon stump.

Less commonly, patients present for evaluation of a closed injury that is associated with loss of finger motion. These patients usually describe loss of distal interphalangeal joint motion following an injury. Patients with a closed tendon avulsion injury may also describe a painful nodule in the area of tendon retraction (usually the palm).

Physical Examination

Patients who have complete flexor tendon injuries will have loss of the normal "flexor cascade" (Fig. 1). Increasing the amount of wrist dorsiflexion will not increase the flexor tone in the fingers with complete tendon injuries. The integrity of tendon can be determined by asking the patient to flex each joint individually. Adjacent finger flexion and proximal joint flexion should be blocked. The location of the laceration(s), two-point discrimination, and capil-

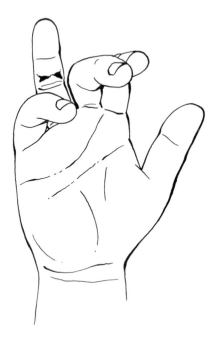

FIG. 1. Loss of the normal flexor cascade after palmar digital laceration.

lary refill should be determined. Allen's test should be performed at the wrist on the digit (Chapter 4, Physical Examination of the Hand).

Carefully palpating the flexor tendon sheath may elicit tenderness proximally at the site of tendon retraction. Patients with a flexor digitorum profundus avulsion injury often have a painful nodule in the palm, which represents the retracted tendon.

A PA and lateral radiograph should be performed when a fracture is suspected.

Palmar digital lacerations should be divided into four general categories based on the physical examination findings: simple lacerations, lacerations with associated tendon injuries, lacerations with associated tendon, nerve and vessel injuries and near amputations.

Painful digital flexion is suggestive of a partial tendon injury. Loss of digital flexion is consistent with a complete tendon transection.

TREATMENT

In general simple lacerations, lacerations with isolated tendon injury and lacerations with associated nerve injuries can receive initial treatment in the emergency room (Chapter 14, Soft-Tissue Injuries and Lacerations). Lacerations associated with significant soft-tissue contamination or lacerations with associated circulatory compromise should be treated on the day of injury.

Initial Treatment

If the digit is well vascularized, then initial care often consists of a wound debridement and closure in the emergency room. Debride and cleanse the wound after establishing satisfactory local or block anesthesia and the application of a tourniquet. Explore the base of the wound to exclude the possibility of an open joint and assess the tendons. Suture the wound with a monofilament nylon suture. Ensure follow-up within 3 to 7 days.

Definitive Treatment

Injuries in zones 3, 4, and 5 (Fig. 2) often require definitive treatment on the day of injury because they are often associated with injury to major nerves and arteries. Injuries that are associated with significant circulatory abnormalities always require treatment on the day of injury.

Formal tendon repair is done in an operating room under regional or general anesthesia. The zone of injury usually influences the method of repair. For injuries within the synovial sheath of the digit (zones 1 and 2) it is important to repair the tendon with a suture method that is strong enough to allow early digital mobilization, but also results in a smooth repair site so that the tendon can glide through the narrow fibroosseous tunnel of the digit. Certain repair methods (multistrand, multigrasp methods) are strong enough to allow early active

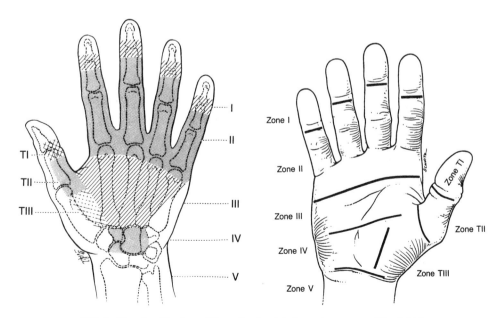

FIG. 2. The classification of flexor tendon injuries using zones of the hand.

digital mobilization. The location of the tendon injury and the method chosen for tendon repair influence the postoperative rehabilitation regimen. Associated repair of nerves and arteries also can be completed at the time of tendon repair.

Partial Tendon Injuries

If the injury is greater than 50% of the cross sectional area of the tendon, then tendon repair is done. Smaller tendon injuries usually can be treated with debridement of the flap and early mobilization. Partial tendon injuries are treated to limit the risk of four complications: rupture, triggering, entrapment, and stiffness.

Flexor Digitorum Profundus Avulsion Injuries

Avulsion of the flexor digitorum profundus is treated by primary tendon advancement and repair when possible. If the patient presents early following injury, then tendon advancement and repair are usually possible. The method of distal tendon fixation is determined by the presence or absence of a fracture. If the fragment represents a significant segment of the joint surface, then an open reduction and internal fixation should be considered.

If patients present after three weeks following injury, primary repair is not possible. For these cases the treatment alternatives include observation, distal interphalangeal joint fusion, distal FDP tenodesis for distal joint stabilization, and tendon graft reconstruction.

After flexor tendon repair, patients are usually immobilized in a specialized splint that positions the wrist in approximately 30 degrees of palmar flexion, the metacarpal phalangeal joints in approximately 70 degrees of palmar flexion, and the interphalangeal joints in mild flexion.

Occupational therapy should be scheduled as soon as possible following the procedure. The type of repair that was done and the ability of the patient to cooperate with the aftercare program influence the specific method of rehabilitation selected.

Often patients require a prolonged period of rehabilitation following tendon repair. If, after 4 months, patients have not regained a satisfactory amount of digital flexion, they should be considered for tenolysis.

KEY POINTS

- Flexor tendon injuries are different from extensor tendon injuries because they usually require formal repair in the operating room.
- Tendon repairs in zones 1 and 2 are the most difficult areas to obtain an excellent patient outcome.
- Flexor pollicis longus lacerations often retract proximally into the distal forearm.

• Definitive repair of the tendon should be done within 10 days of injury. Flexor digitorum profundus avulsion injuries should be treated early to increase the chances of primary flexor tendon repair.

SELECTED REFERENCES

Gelberman RH, Nunley JA, Osterman AL, Breen TF, Dimick MP, Woo SLY. Influences of the protected passive mobilization interval on flexor tendon healing: a prospective randomized clinical study. Clin Orthop 1991;264:189–196.

Strickland JW. Flexor tendon injuries: foundations of treatment. J Am Acad Orthop Surg 1995;3:44–54.

Strickland JW. Flexor tendon injuries: operative technique. J Am Acad Orthop Surg 1995;3:55–62.

17

Nerve Injuries

GENERAL INFORMATION

The median, ulnar, and radial nerves are the terminal branches of the brachial plexus and supply motor, sensory, and sympathetic function to the hand (Appendix 4, Radial, Ulnar, and Median Nerve Anatomy). Hand surgeons commonly evaluate both acute and chronic nerve conditions.

NERVE LACERATIONS

Diagnostic Criteria

Most peripheral nerve lacerations occur following a penetrating injury (e.g., glass or knife wounds).

History

Patients with median nerve lacerations describe numbness in the thumb, index, long, and ring fingers, and weakness of thumb abduction. Those with ulnar nerve lacerations complain of numbness in the ring and small fingers and have clawing of the ring and small fingers. Those with radial nerve lacerations have weakness of wrist, finger, and digital extension and decreased feeling in the web space between the thumb and index finger.

Physical Examination

Most patients have a Tinel's sign at the sight of nerve injury. Detailed physical examination shows a neurologic deficit in the distribution of the involved peripheral nerve.

TREATMENT

Surgical exploration using optical magnification allows anatomic coaptation of the nerve ends. Most repairs approximate the outer layer (epineurium) of the nerve after alignment of interval nerve fibers (fascicles). Epineural repairs also help prevent disorderly growth of new axons (neuromas). Large nerve gaps require nerve grafting.

AFTERCARE

Splint protection of nerve repair is necessary for 3 to 4 weeks. Functional bracing permits proper hand position while motor axons regenerate. Hand therapy is often beneficial.

RESULTS

Microsurgical repairs result in varying return of function based on age and level of laceration, mechanism of injury, the specific nerve involved, and individual health status. Following a laceration, the distal nerve undergoes wallerian degeneration and must be replaced by new axons growing across the repair site. After 30 days, peripheral nerves regenerate at 1 mm per day. Clinically, an "advancing Tinel's sign" is consistent with nerve regeneration.

NERVE COMPRESSION

Nerve compression occurs when increased pressure on a peripheral nerve results in local ischemia and decreased axonal transport. Early symptoms are pain and paresthesias. As compression worsens, patients develop fixed (constant) numbness, loss of dexterity, and weakness.

CARPAL TUNNEL SYNDROME

Carpal tunnel syndrome, or compression of the median nerve beneath the transverse carpal ligament and is the most common entrapment neuropathy.

DIAGNOSTIC CRITERIA

History

Patients describe numbness and tingling in the thumb, index, long, and half of the ring finger. Numbness and pain are worse at night, often causing nocturnal awakening. Daytime activities, such as driving with the wrists extended, may exacerbate the symptoms. Clumsiness and weakness of grip are also common complaints. Pain usually occurs in the distal volar forearm and hand.

Carpal tunnel syndrome is more common in women, and in patients with diabetes mellitus, and rheumatoid arthritis. Other associated conditions are listed in Table 1.

TABLE 1. *Conditions associated with carpal tunnel syndrome*

Diabetes
Flexor tenosynovitis
Gout
Hypothyroidism
Lipoma
Renal failure and dialysis
Obesity
Thrombosis of median artery

Physical Examination

Physical examination for carpal tunnel begins by excluding other sources of nerve compression (brachial plexopathy and proximal median nerve compression). Tinel's test, Phalen's maneuver, and Durkan's test are usually positive. A reverse Phalen's maneuver, with the wrist hyperextended, should produce similar symptoms. Direct compression over the median nerve reproducing numbness in the median nerve distribution is a sensitive and specific test for carpal tunnel syndrome (Durkan's test). Patients with moderate to severe involvement will have abnormalities on two-point discrimination (2PD) and Semmes-Weinstein monofilament testing. Weakness and abductor pollicis brevis atrophy are suggestive of severe involvement.

The diagnosis of carpal tunnel syndrome is confirmed using standardized electrodiagnostic testing (Fig. 1).

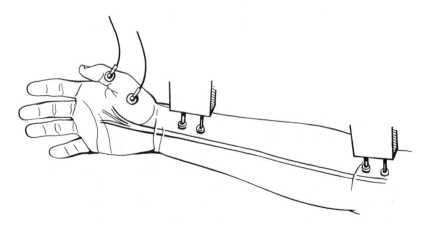

FIG. 1. Electrodiagnostic testing.

TREATMENT

Initial treatment of carpal tunnel syndrome employs wrist splinting and the use of nonsteroidal antiinflammatory drugs. Activity modification and therapeutic exercises also may improve symptoms. These treatments are most effective within the first 3 to 6 months of symptom onset.

The next step in treatment is injection of the carpal canal. Steroid injections into the carpal canal have been shown to decrease symptoms in 80% to 90% of patients for 3 to 9 months. During this time of relief, the results "mimic" the results of surgical intervention and are a good preview if surgery is considered later.

Technique for Carpal Canal Injection (Fig. 2)

- Prepare a sterile solution of 1-mL 1% Xylocaine and 1-mL water-soluble steroid medication (i.e., dexamethasone, sodium phosphate) in a 3-mL syringe with a 25-gauge 1½-in. needle.
- Complete a sterile preparation of the skin.
- Insert the needle into the wrist flexor crease at a 45-degree angle to the skin in line with the ring finger metacarpal.

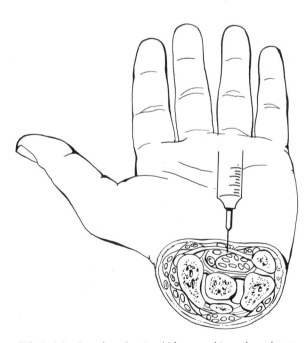

FIG. 2. Injection of corticosteroid for carpal tunnel syndrome.

- Insert the needle to the floor of the carpal canal and withdraw the needle slightly.
- The solution may be injected if the patient is not experiencing paresthesias.
- Apply a Bandaid.

Surgical treatment usually results in significant improvement of the symptoms of carpal tunnel syndrome. Open carpal tunnel release is the standard against which all other modalities are measured.

CUBITAL TUNNEL SYNDROME

Compression of the ulnar nerve at the elbow is the second most common entrapment neuropathy in the upper extremity. The ulnar nerve is posterior and inferior to the medial epicondyle of the elbow and medial to the olecranon. Both traction and compression have been implicated in causing cubital tunnel syndrome. Superficial to the nerve is a fibrous band, Osborne's ligament, which tightens with elbow flexion and may lead to external compression. Occasionally, the ligament is incompetent or lax and allows subluxation of the nerve anteriorly (snapping ulnar nerve). The nerve is subject to mechanical traction with elbow flexion, which may further exacerbate disruption of microcirculation and lead to symptoms.

DIAGNOSTIC CRITERIA

History

Patients with cubital tunnel syndrome present with numbness and tingling predominantly in the ring and small fingers. Discomfort on the medial side of the elbow and complaints of pain in the "funny bone" are also common descriptions. Often a history of bumping the elbow or remote elbow fracture is elicited. People who sleep with the elbows flexed are also at risk.

Physical Examination

Provocative maneuvers include Tinel's testing in the groove posterior to the medial epicondyle. The elbow flexion test places the elbow in flexion, the forearm in supination, and the wrist extended (waiter's position). A positive test reproduces numbness and tingling in the ulnar digits. Sensory testing should include both the palmar and dorsal aspect of the ring and small fingers. This helps differentiate compression at the elbow from compression at the wrist as the dorsal sensory nerve branches proximal to the wrist.

Clawing of the ring and small fingers (hyperextension of the metaphalangeal joints with flexion of the interphalangeal joints) is a classic finding of severe ulnar neuropathy.

Electrodiagnostic studies are helpful in discriminating cubital tunnel from other neurologic condition.

TREATMENT

Nonoperative treatment focuses on limiting nerve traction and nerve contact. Daytime splinting, using a heel-so or other posterior elbow pad, is helpful in reducing symptoms, especially in early cases. Pillow splints may prevent flexion and improve symptoms at night.

Surgical decompression of the nerve is indicated for refractory numbness and weakness, especially if atrophy is present. Techniques vary, but results are good in up to 80% of cases. Recovery is slower than after carpal tunnel surgery, and patients with advanced changes or diabetes may have incomplete symptom resolution. Occupational therapy is indicated for elbow stiffness, scar tenderness, and sensitivity. Other common nerve compressions are listed in Table 2.

TABLE 2. *Other peripheral entrapment neuropathies*

Nerve involvement	Level of initial neuropathy	Signs and symptoms	Treatment
Saturday night palsy of the radial nerve	Posterior mid- to distal humerus "spiral groove"	Common radial nerve palsy Numbness first web	Rest NSAID Splint
Radial tunnel	Proximal dorsoradial forearm	Posterior interosseous nerve palsy Pain in forearm worse with resisted supination	Rest NSAID injection
Wartenberg's neuritis Superficial radial nerve	Distal forearm 10 cm proximal to radial styloid	Numbness in first web space Tinel's over superficial radial nerve	Splint NSAID
Pronator syndrome (median nerve)	Proximal medial forearm	Numbness thumb-ring and proximal palm Hypertrophic pronator muscle	Rest Stretching exercises Surgery
Anterior interosseous nerve palsy	Forearm	Isolation palsy of the FPL; FDP index	Rest NSAID
Ulnar tunnel	Wrist Guyon's canal	Mass in ulnar palm Intrinsic weakness/ atrophy Tinel's at canal	Rest Splint NSAID

FDP, flexor digitorum profundus; *FPL,* flexor pollicis longus. *NSAID,* nonsteroidal antiinflammatory drug.

SELECTED REFERENCES

Phalen GS, et al. Neuropathy of the median nerve due to compression beneath the transverse carpal ligament. J Bone Joint Surg 1950;32A:109–112.

Hadler NM. Occupational illness: the issue of causality. J Occup Med 1984;26:587–593.

Louis D. Evaluation and treatment of median neuropathy associated with cumulative trauma. In: Gelberman RH, ed. Operative nerve repair and reconstruction. Lippincott, Philadelphia, 1991, p. 957–961.

Durkan JA. A new diagnostic test for carpal tunnel syndrome. J Bone Joint Surg 1991;73A:112–117.

18

Arterial Injuries

GENERAL INFORMATION

Significant redundancy exists in the vascular supply to the upper extremity. The brachial artery has radial and ulnar collateral vessels at the elbow. The radial and ulnar arteries form a parallel inflow system that may be accompanied by a deep interosseous artery in the forearm. Two palmar arches supply the wrist and hand. Each digit has two palmar arteries and a variable dorsal outflow system. These vessels are superficial at the medial elbow, distal volar forearm, and palmar aspect of the digit. Lacerations that violate the fascia at these levels should lead to suspicion of arterial injury even if inflow exists. Arteries have muscular walls, which decrease blood loss by going into spasm when injured. This same property retracts the cut ends of the vessel from the zone of injury making the diagnosis more difficult. In contrast, partially injured vessels, especially those with longitudinal tears, may bleed freely and present with ongoing pulsatile blood loss.

DIAGNOSTIC CRITERIA

Patients with arterial injuries distal to the elbow may present as lacerations with sudden, dramatic blood loss and distal ischemia. These injuries are not difficult to diagnose and require prompt treatment to minimize tissue loss and systemic complications. Patients with these injuries may also present more subtly with a laceration or puncture, which bleeds briefly, then stops. A high index of suspicion and complete workup confirm the diagnosis and prevent late symptoms of pain, exercise, and cold intolerance, or even tissue loss.

Emergency treatment of arterial bleeding involves control of the blood vessel. Distal to the elbow, direct pressure over a lacerated vessel generally controls blood loss. This is initially applied as direct pressure and later supplemented by a compressive bandage. In severe cases, a pneumatic tourniquet or blood pressure cuff inflation proximal to the injury stems blood flow. Cuff pressure should be 50 to 100 mm Hg above systolic blood pressure (Fig. 1). These injuries require emergency evaluation by a specialist who can undertake arterial repair.

135

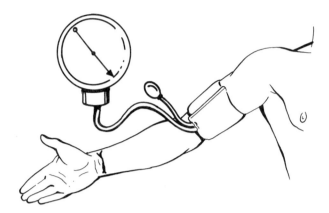

FIG. 1. The use of a pressure cuff to control bleeding. This method can be used to temporarily control bleeding while additional evaluation and emergency consultation is obtained.

Random probing and clamping in uncontrolled bleeding may lead to nerve injury because nervous and arterial structures lie in close proximity to each other throughout the forearm and hand.

History

A history of the injury is obtained once bleeding is controlled. Glass lacerations may produce an innocuous-appearing skin wound with significant deep vessel, nerve, and tendon injury. Sensibility and movement of the injured extremity helps identify other injured structures. Distal signs of ischemia include a pale, pulseless digit or extremity. This can be conveniently evaluated by pulse oximetry. Loss of oximetry signals with all tourniquet compression removed is an indication for urgent exploration and repair. Such injuries are deemed "critical" and can occur when both neurovascular bundles are lacerated in the digit or both radial and ulnar arteries are lacerated in the forearm. These injuries require emergent surgical exploration and repair. Normal oximetry values suggest that distal perfusion is adequate.

Physical Examination

Simple palpation of peripheral pulses is not adequate to exclude arterial injury. Pulse waves may be transmitted even in the absence of flow, especially in diabetics and those with atherosclerotic peripheral vascular disease. Retrograde flow from an intact vessel may also produce pulsations. Assessing capillary refill does not preclude arterial injury. The Allen's test, however, is sensitive for single vessel injury in the forearm. Occluding both the radial and ulnar vessels while the patient flexes and extends the fingers performs the test. This creates pallor in palm and digits. Release of pressure on either radial or ulnar vessel should allow return of normal color within 2 to 5 seconds. Failure to restore flow to the digits after release of radial pressure indicates arterial occlusion or laceration on the ulnar side and vice versa. Side-to-side comparisons are performed to detect subtle changes and rule out congenitally incomplete vascular arches. The test can be performed to evaluate digital flow as well.

Doppler studies including standard ultrasonic probes or visual duplex probes are important adjuncts to physical examination in diagnosis of arterial injury. Arteriography represents the gold standard of blood flow assessment. Arteriography remains crucial in evaluating thromboembolic disease. Routine x-rays are useful for detecting foreign bodies associated with penetrating trauma but not vessel injuries. Magnetic resonance angiography is useful in congenital vascular disorders or posttraumatic anomalies, but not in acute injury evaluation.

TREATMENT

Absolute indications for arterial repair include uncontrolled bleeding and distal ischemia. Reperfusion of the upper extremity relieves pain and restores motor function. Prolonged ischemia (>4 to 6 hours) leads to significant muscular swelling and may lead to compartment syndrome. Prophylactic fasciotomy is performed, especially in cases where the patient may be obtunded. Relative indications for vascular repair include associated nerve or tendon injuries requiring surgical repair. Isolated digital or forearm vessel repair remains controversial. Traditionally, backflow from the distal segment of a lacerated vessel indicated adequate flow and repairs not undertaken. Repair patency rates were only 10% to 20% prior to development of microsurgical techniques. Newer microvascular techniques, however, result in 80% patency rates when performed shortly after the injury. Collateral vessels form over time if the repair is not performed.

Complications of unrepaired vessels include formation of an arteriovenous fistula or aneurysm. Presenting as a pulsatile mass at the site of previous trauma, these may be asymptomatic or cause distal ischemia from embolization of clots from an aneurysm. Arteriovenous fistulas shunt blood away from distal capillary beds and can cause ischemia, ulcer formation, or exercise intolerance. Symptomatic lesions require excision and repair or grafting of the injured artery.

INTRAARTERIAL INJECTIONS

Intraarterial injections remain a potentially devastating arterial injury, often leading to digital or hand necrosis and amputation. Drug injections produce a chemical inflammation of the vessels. Particulate matter embolizes distally, causing vascular occlusion and distal vasospasm. Early intervention with anticoagulation, sympathetic blocks, and occasionally, venous bypass of specific occlusions may improve outcome, especially if the injection occurs in a hospital setting. Unfortunately, many injuries are not treated acutely, especially in recreational drug users. Supportive treatment and eventual amputation of necrotic digits remain the treatment of choice in late presentations.

CANNULATION INJURIES

Arterial cannulation is a common procedure for pressure monitoring, angiographic studies, and blood sampling. The radial artery at the wrist is a common site for indwelling catheters. Prior to insertion of a radial artery catheter, the Allen's test will reveal obstructions of ulnar artery flow that preclude insertion of a radial-sided cannula. The catheter itself can injure the vessel lumen and cause thrombosis, embolization, and possibly ischemia. Aneurysm formation may occur after the catheter is removed and dissection occurs between arterial walls layers. If vascular compromise occurs following catheter insertion, then remove the catheter quickly, which may restore flow. Significant compromise suggests a need for thrombectomy and possibly arterial reconstruction.

SELECTED REFERENCES

Lee RE, et al. Acute penetrating arterial injuries of the forearm: ligation or repair? Am Surg 1985;51: 318–384.
Taras JS, Lemel MS, Nathan R. Vascular disorders of the upper extremity. In: Hunter, et al. Rehabilitation of the hand: surgery and therapy, 4th ed. Mosby, Philadelphia, 1978.
Wilgis EF, ed. Vascular disorders. WB Saunders, Philadelphia, 1993.

19

Vascular Disorders

EVALUATION

Many patients with vascular disorders complain of pain and color changes of the hand. Pallor and coolness indicate loss of inflow, whereas redness and cyanosis indicate loss of outflow. Patients may note increased symptoms in cold weather. A history of blunt or penetrating trauma, vibratory tool use, tobacco use, and a past medical history of arrhythmias or connective tissue disease should be sought.

On examination, the color and temperature of the finger should be noted. The fingertip is examined for ulcers or splinter hemorrhages. Palpation and a Doppler test measure peripheral pulses. An Allen's test is done to determine the patency of the radial and ulnar arterial supply to the fingers.

VASCULAR DISORDERS

Thrombosis

Thrombosis of the ulnar artery at Guyon's canal (hypothenar hammer syndrome) is the most common thrombosis in the hand. It is usually secondary to repeated blunt trauma to the hypothenar eminence. Patients complain of a tender mass in the region. The mass often compresses the ulnar nerve in Guyon's canal, giving numbness to the small finger and ulnar border of the ring finger. Ischemia of the ring and small fingers may develop from emboli, vasospasm, or an incomplete arch. Examination is noted for an Allen's test that shows no flow through the ulnar artery and a tender mass in Guyon's canal. Treatment consists of cessation of smoking and initiation of vasodilators, such as calcium channel blockers. The thrombosed segment may require surgical excision with reconstruction. Transection of the segment improves digital blood supply by interrupting the sympathetic nerve fibers to the fingers. Reconstruction of the involved segment improves blood supply to the hand.

Thrombosis of the radial or ulnar arteries also may come from an inadvertent intraarterial injection. Patients usually complain of immediate and intense burning pain. The spasm can lead to thrombosis and occlusion of the vessels. Initial treatment consists of vasodilators, a sympathetic nerve block, and either anticoagulants or systemic thrombolytic therapy. If an isolated clot is present proximally, thrombectomy or excision and grafting of the involved segment may be helpful. The outcome is often related to the agent that was injected.

Aneurysm

There are two types of aneurysms. True aneurysms involve the intima, media, and adventitia. They are usually secondary to blunt trauma. They are likely to produce distal emboli. False aneurysms come from penetrating trauma or arterial perforations. The periarterial hematoma endothelializes and forms a false wall. A painful, pulsatile mass is often present on physical examination. A thrill may be present with palpation over the mass.

Resection of the aneurysm is recommended to prevent thrombosis and emboli. Vascular reconstruction may be necessary depending on the intraoperative examination of the fingers.

Embolus

The upper extremity receives 15% to 20% of all arterial emboli. Mural thrombi from atrial fibrillation, myocardial infarction, and heart valves account for 70% of upper extremity emboli. Large thrombi often lodge at the brachial bifurcation. The patient notes sudden limb pain and ischemia. Treatment consists of an embolectomy.

Microemboli are usually arterial in origin and originate from upper extremity aneurysms or atherosclerotic regions. Patients may experience intermittent embolic showers into one extremity. Treatment consists of identifying and treating the source, reversal of secondary vasospasm, thrombolytic therapy and anticoagulation.

VASOSPASTIC DISORDERS

Raynaud's phenomenon is seen as a triple color change of the digit. The fingers become white from ischemia with cold exposure or emotional distress. The fingers may then turn cyanotic from some venous filling. Finally, as the fingers are warmed, they turn red from vasodilation and hyperemia.

Primary vasospastic disorder, formerly known as Raynaud's disease, is the occurrence of Raynaud's phenomenon without a demonstrable associative or causative disease. It mainly involves both arms in young women. Gangrene or trophic changes are limited to the distal fingertips.

Secondary vasospastic disorder, formerly known as Raynaud's syndrome, is associated with or caused by a disease. The most common association is connective tissue disorders, with 90% of patients in this category having sclero-derma. Other conditions include neurologic disorders, arteriooclusive disorders, blood dyscrasias, and frostbite.

The diagnosis of vasospastic disorder is made by a cold stress test. Digital plethysmography, or digital pulse volume recording, is done before and after cold immersion of the fingers. A sympathetic block is given and the pressures remeasured to determine if the decreased blood flow is sympathetically mediated.

Treatment includes protection of fingers from cold (wear mittens instead of gloves) and trauma. Patients must stop all caffeine and tobacco use. Biofeedback is helpful in some patients. Oral medications include calcium channel blockers (nifedipine) and platelet antagonists such as aspirin. Nitroglycerin ointment may be applied locally to the fingers to provide an alpha receptor blockade and vessel dilation. Palmar and/or digital sympathetectomies may be helpful when pulse volume recordings show improvement following a sympathetic block.

CONGENITAL VASCULAR GROWTHS

Hemangioma

The natural history of a hemangioma is absence at birth, quick growth after birth, and slow involution. Of all hemangiomas, 70% are gone by age 7 years. The female to male ratio is 3:1. Treatment should be reassurance and local wound care.

Low-Flow Vascular Malformations

A capillary malformation, "port wine stain," is a collection of dilated capillaries and venules in the upper dermis. A venous malformation, formerly called a cavernous hemangioma, is present at birth. It has a slow, steady rate of growth. This lesion is compressible. Magnetic resonance imaging will confirm it to be a low-flow vascular growth.

When the lesions are discrete, they may be excised if symptomatic. When diffuse, careful preoperative planning is required to understand the major vessels feeding the mass. It is often helpful to stage excision of large masses, removing all that can be excised from a single incision.

High-Flow Vascular Malformations

Arteriovenous malformations are multiple large or small fistulas that divert blood flow from feeding arteries to draining veins. They lead to proximal venous dilatation and hypertrophy. Distally, they produce an arterial steal and ischemia. On examination, a thrill is palpable in the draining veins.

Treatment of the lesions is controversial. Some authors recommend excising symptomatic lesions only. Embolization of the arteriovenous malformations may be helpful.

SELECTED REFERENCE

American Society for Surgery of the Hand, ed. 1998 Regional review courses in hand surgery. American Society for Surgery of the Hand, Rosemont, IL, 1998, pp. 3-1 – 3-17.

20

Dermatologic Disorders

GENERAL EXAMINATION

Examination of the skin is an extremely important part of the evaluation of the upper extremity. The clinician should note the overall appearance, texture, and color, as well as the presence of any skin lesions, rash, nicotine stains, and nail abnormalities. The way the hand has been used can be determined by the presence or absence of calluses on the palm and fingers.

DIFFERENTIAL DIAGNOSIS

The appearance of the skin can give the physician clues as to the underlying disease process. For example, in reflex sympathetic dystrophy the skin may have abnormal sweating, appear shiny, and lose its normal wrinkled appearance. After a nerve transection, the skin becomes dry and there is a demonstrable loss of sweat in the sensory dermatomal distribution of the injured nerve.

Skin ulcers can be seen at the tips of the digits in conditions associated with ischemia (i.e., scleroderma, Buerger's disease, Raynaud's disease, and Crest syndrome) (Fig. 1).

Scleroderma is associated with fingers that become slender, shiny, and immobile (metaphalangeal [MP] extension contractures and proximal interphalangeal [PIP] flexion contractures). Skin breakdown and ulcers are common in areas where the skin is stretched, such as over the dorsum of the proximal interphalangeal joints with PIP flexion contractures (Fig. 2).

It is important to note any evidence of psoriasis, which may include a scaly, erythematous skin rash over extensor surfaces of the elbow and several other areas of the body. Typical nail findings in psoriasis include pitting and crumbling. Approximately 5% of patients with psoriasis have an inflammatory arthritis, and 15% to 20% of patients develop the skin lesions after the onset of arthritis. Isolated proximal interphalangeal joint swelling is commonly seen with psoriatic arthritis. Psoriatic arthritis, unlike rheumatoid arthritis, can be asymmetric (Fig. 3). Osteolysis at the distal interphalangeal (DIP) joints results in a "pencil in cup" appearance.

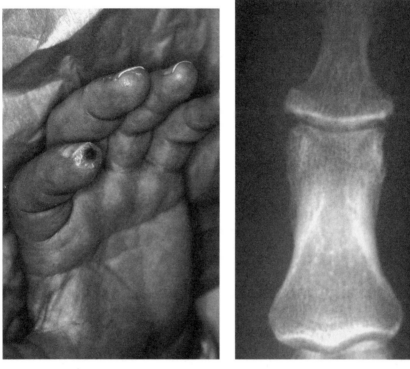

FIG. 1. A: Unhealing ischemic ulcer at tip of index finger in an individual with CREST syndrome. **B:** X-ray showing chronic osteomyelitis at tip of distal phalanx.

ONYCHOMYCOSIS

Fungal infections of the nail, most commonly seen in the toes, can also be seen in the fingers (Fig. 4). Predisposing factors include heat, moisture, trauma, false nails, diabetes, inheritance, aging, and altered immunologic status. The diagnosis can be confirmed by a potassium hydroxide (KOH) preparation from the nail clippings or subungual keratotic debris.

Treatment

A combined surgical and medical approach may be indicated. The diseased nail can be cut back or completely removed and the underlying nail bed curetted in an attempt to debulk the fungus. Several topical preparations have been used with limited, temporary success. Lamisil cream (terbinafine hydrochloride 1%) has been the most effective and should be applied for 2 to 3 months. Oral griseofulvin was used in the past. Pulsed treatment of oral Sporanox (itraconazole) is recommended: 200 mg bid for 1 week separated by a 3-week period, followed by

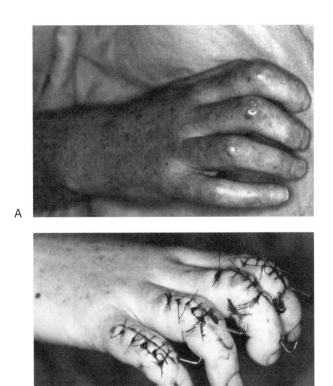

FIG. 2. A: A woman with scleroderma with metaphalangeal extension contractures and PIP flexion contractures. Note skin breakdown over dorsum of proximal interphalangeal (PIP) joints. **B:** Treatment with multiple PIP fusions in a more extended position.

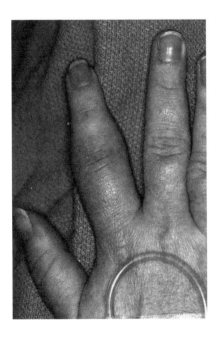

FIG. 3. Early psoriatic arthritis with unilateral isolated involvement in the proximal interphalangeal joint of the index finger.

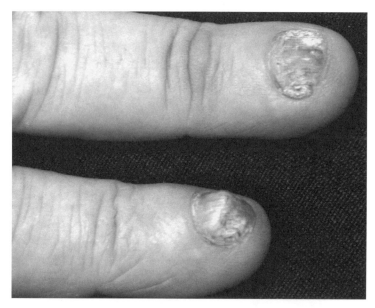

FIG. 4. Untreated onychomycosis.

1 more week of treatment. (Pulsed treatment is not recommended when treating the toes.)

PYOGENIC GRANULOMA

Seen in all ages and in all areas of the body, a pyogenic granuloma is a proliferating capillary hemangioma that usually arises at the site of minor trauma (Fig. 5). Early small lesions are bright red, lobulated, and friable, resulting in considerable bleeding if irritated. The lesions rarely exceed 1 cm and may turn brown, yellow, or black with time, and manifest a purulent exudate.

Treatment

Marginal excision or curettage and electrodesiccation have been most successful. Serial application of silver nitrate is adequate for smaller lesions.

SKIN LESIONS

Many diverse tumors are associated with the skin. Signs of malignancy may include continuous growth, ulceration, marked deformity, odor, enlargement, and firmness. These are frequently treated initially as an infection. Any lesions that do not heal properly should raise suspicion for malignancy.

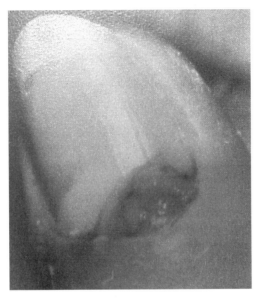

FIG. 5. Pyogenic granuloma arising from the base of the thumb nail.

KERATOACANTHOMA

A keratoacanthoma (KA) is a common lesion of the hand. This tumor appears in sun-exposed areas in middle-aged and older patients as an elevated papular growth. The lesion may reach up to 2 cm or more in diameter within 2 to 4 weeks. A crater develops with a core of keratinous material. These lesions grow rapidly. Keratoacanthoma, similar to squamous cell carcinoma, develops in skin that has been exposed to radiation, chemical exposure, and scarring, and can be seen in immunocompromised individuals (Fig. 6).

Treatment

In general, biopsy of any questionable skin lesion is mandatory. Excision is recommended once the diagnosis of keratoacanthoma is established.

SQUAMOUS CELL CARCINOMA

Squamous cell carcinomas are the most common malignant tumors in the hand. They may appear to be slow-growing wartlike lesions or may become large, ulcerated, and exophytic (Fig. 7). Squamous cell carcinomas can spread locally and metastasize using lymphatic or hematogenous routes.

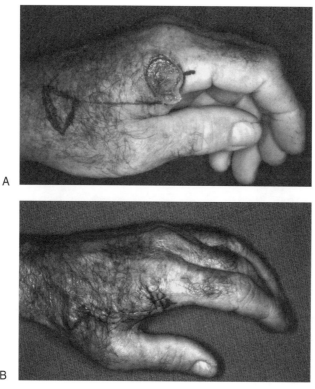

FIG. 6. A: Keratoacanthosis at the base of the index finger. **B:** Treatment with excision and rotational flap closure.

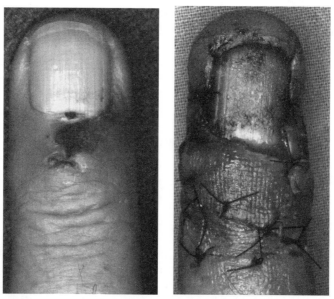

FIG. 7. A: Squamous cell carcinoma *in situ* (Bowen's disease), status post biopsy after presentation with an erythematous ulcerated lesion at the base of the nail. **B:** Treatment with excision, rotation flap closure, and skin grafting.

Treatment

Treatment consists of wide excision after the diagnosis is confirmed by biopsy. These patients usually need evaluation by a medical oncologist for adjuvant treatment. An orthopedic oncologist should also evaluate some patients.

MALIGNANT MELANOMA

The incidence of malignant melanoma is increasing in the United States. A significant number of malignant melanomas arise in the sun-exposed skin of the upper limb. Malignant lesions may arise from a melanocytic nevus. Benign lesions are well circumscribed and evenly pigmented. Any existing lesion that shows a change or a lesion with irregular borders, a variation of pigmentation (red, white, or blue) or ulceration, should be biopsied.

Several types of melanomas exist. Acral-lentiginous melanoma refers to a melanoma involving the palms of the hands or the nailbed areas (Fig. 8). These develop relatively rapidly and occur often in older patients. They may be associated with a variety of colors. They can present as flat, pigmented lesions with irregular borders or as a mass with an overlying ulcer. A delay in diagnosis is common because these lesions are frequently mistaken for warts, paronychias, or chronic ulcers.

Subungual melanomas manifest with a colored streak down the nail, which can be difficult to diagnose in African Americans, and must be differentiated from a subungual hematoma or infection.

Treatment

Treatment consists of a wide resection, after confirmation by biopsy. A workup for regional lymph node spread and metastasis to other organs is indicated. Chemotherapy and immunotherapy regimens are often indicated. Patients benefit from referral to a medical oncologist for evaluation and treatment.

EPITHELIOID SARCOMA

Epithelioid sarcoma is a slow-growing malignancy of uncertain cell origin that is commonly found in the upper extremities, frequently on the palmar surface of the hand and digits, in 20- to 40-year-old individuals. It usually appears as an inflammatory reaction in the skin that can cause pain and tenderness leading to ulceration; it may seem to be an infection, although it may appear simply as a small mass. Clinically, the underlying mass is firm and immobile as a result of adherence to surrounding tissues. Metastasis is by lymphatic as well as hematogenous spread. Magnetic resonance imaging prior to biopsy is indicated (Fig. 9).

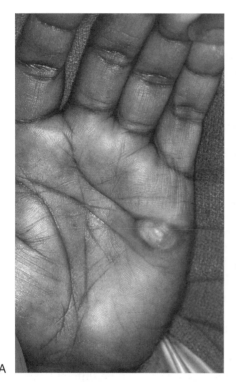

A

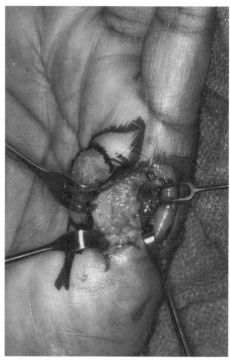

B

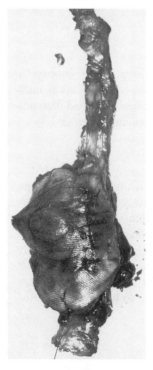

C

FIG. 8. A: Malignant melanoma in the palm (Acral-lentiginous melanoma). Initially mistaken for a nonhealing skin lesion with callus formation. **B:** Open biopsy of lesion. **C:** Definitive treatment with ray resection. Concomitant lymph node dissection showed spread to epitrochlear and axillary nodes.

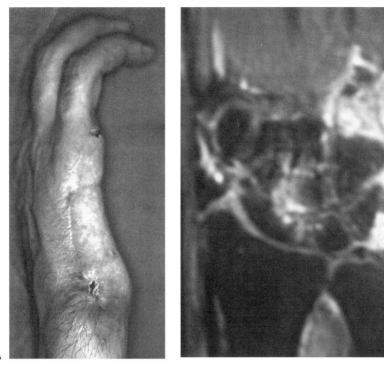

A   B

FIG. 9. A: Status post ray resection for an epithelioid sarcoma, presenting 1 year later with small nonhealing ulcer at the edge of previous resection site. **B:** Magnetic resonance imaging scan showing underlying recurrent lesion.

Treatment

The treatment is wide excision and possibly radiation. No effective chemotherapy is currently available. Referral to a medical oncologist is indicated.

KEY POINTS

- Suspicious skin lesions, including nonhealing ulcers, should undergo biopsy.
- Patients who present with malignant lesions benefit from multidisciplinary evaluation and treatment. Early referral to a medical oncologist will help organize the patient's care. A musculoskeletal oncologist or surgical oncologist is often helpful in tailoring patient treatment pathways.

SELECTED REFERENCES

Scher RK, Daniel. Nails: therapy, diagnosis, surgery. WB Saunders, Philadelphia, 1990.
Tumors of the hand and forearm. Hand Clin 1987;3:2.

21

Infections

FELON

General Information

A felon is a deep infection of the finger pulp (Fig. 1), and accounts for approximately 15% of hand infections. There is usually a history of a puncture wound or an open injury to the digit. *Staphylococcus aureus* is the usual causative organism. The infection is trapped between the vertical septae that divide the pulp and stabilize the skin.

DIAGNOSTIC CRITERIA

Clinically, the patient has a throbbing pain at the tip of the digit. The pain and swelling can develop quickly. The pulp is tightly swollen, tender, and erythematous. Purulence may be present. Cultures of any purulent material should be taken. One should look for the potential complications of an untreated felon, including osteomyelitis of the distal phalanx, pyogenic arthritis of the distal interphalangeal joint, flexor tenosynovitis, and skin necrosis.

X-rays of the finger should be taken to rule out the presence of a foreign body or distal phalangeal osteomyelitis.

TREATMENT

Nonoperative treatment may be used in treating an early felon with mild swelling or infection that is already adequately draining. Nonoperative treatment includes the use of warm soaks, intensive local wound care, oral antibiotics, and careful follow-up.

Operative treatment is used in treating a felon with moderate or severe symptoms, the presence of osteomyelitis, septic arthritis, or flexor tenosynovitis. Treatment should then include incision and drainage of the felon. A unilateral longitudinal incision is made near the nail skin margin. The incision may be extended to the tip of the digit (Fig. 2). Radial border incisions are made on the

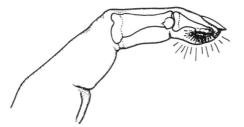

FIG. 1. Felon.

thumb and little fingers. Ulnar border incisions are made on the index and long fingers. Either radial or ulnar border incisions can be made on the ring finger. If the abscess presents in the digital pulp, then an incision may be made in that area (Fig. 3). The vertical fibrous septae within the pulp should be fully divided to ensure that the felon is completely drained. Care should be taken not to cross the flexion creases at a right angle or violate the flexor tendon sheath. The wound should be left open and packed with a small sterile gauze wick. Flexor tenosynovitis or septic arthritis should also be adequately débrided. Any infected bone should be removed. A partial digital amputation may be needed for chronic osteomyelitis. Daily dressing changes should be performed. Warm soaks or whirlpool treatment may be needed.

Cultures should be taken. Antistaphylococcal antibiotics (e.g., penicillinase-resistant penicillin or cephalosporins) usually are given. Antibiotic coverage may need to be changed, depending on the lack of clinical improvement and sensitivities of the cultured bacteria. The antibiotics should be used for an adequate

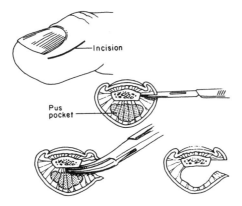

FIG. 2. Drainage of a felon using a midlateral incision. Complete division of the vertical septae should be performed.

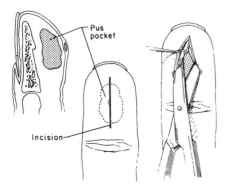

FIG. 3. Drainage of a felon through the pulp.

enough time to allow for clinical improvement. Six weeks of intravenous antibiotics may be needed to treat osteomyelitis.

PARONYCHIA

General Information

A paronychia is an infection that involves the soft tissues around the fingernail (Fig. 4). If the eponychial fold is involved, the infection is referred to as an eponychia, and if the infection invades beneath the nail as well, it is called a subungual abscess.

The usual causative organism is *Staphylococcus aureus* that has been introduced into the paronychial tissue by some trauma (e.g., manicure, a sharp corner of a nail, or a hangnail). In children, thumb sucking can introduce mouth flora and produce an infection. In early stages, the infection may only be superficial to the nail; it may later extend around the border of the nail into the subungual space, resulting in nail destruction; still later, it may invade bone and cause osteomyelitis.

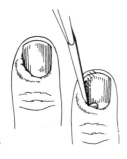

A,B

FIG. 4. A: Paronychia. **B:** Techniques of drainage.

Diagnostic Criteria

A history of precipitating trauma, increasing tenderness, erythema, swelling, and pain is usually noted. Clinically, localized swelling alongside the nail to generalized swelling of the entire distal portion of the distal phalanx in severe cases is seen. The early signs include diffuse inflammation and later abscess formation with fluctuation. Purulence may be present. Cultures of any purulent material should be taken. A herpetic whitlow (see the following), characterized by painful, clear vesicle formation, should be excluded. These infections are reported in health care workers whose hands are in contact with mouth flora (e.g., dentists and anesthesiologists).

X-rays of the finger should be taken to rule out the presence of a foreign body or distal phalangeal osteomyelitis.

Treatment

Nonoperative treatment is used in treating early paronychia with mild swelling or infection that is already adequately draining. Treatment options include trimming of a hangnail or sharp border of a nail, frequent hand washings and/or soaks, and antistaphylococcal antibiotics.

Operative treatment is used in treating paronychia with moderate or severe symptoms, a subungual abscess, felon, or osteomyelitis. Care is taken to apply the digital block proximal to the area of infection. Treatment options include incisional drainage with or without nail plate removal. Elevating the nail margin can drain the abscess (Fig. 4).

In larger more extensive lesions, partial nail removal and/or incision of the nail fold can be performed (Fig. 5).

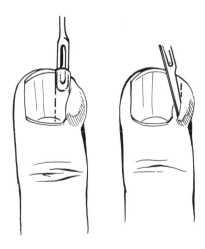

FIG. 5. Drainage of a paronychia with and without a partial nail plate removal.

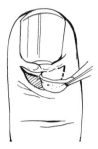

FIG. 6. Drainage of a eponychia.

If an eponychia is present, an incision or incisions into the paronychium, extending into the eponychium (Fig. 6), with or without nail plate excision may be needed.

A subungual abscess is débrided following either partial or complete nail removal. A felon should be adequately drained. A chronic paronychia may be seen in those with occupational exposure to cleaning solutions (e.g., kitchen personnel, housekeepers). Cultures of the infected area in these situations will often be positive for fungus and multiple bacterial organisms. Treatment may require nail removal, marsupialization of the eponychial fold (Fig. 7), and oral antibiotics and topical antifungal ointment. Any infected bone also should be removed. A partial digital amputation may be needed for chronic osteomyelitis.

Cultures should be taken if antibiotics are needed. Warm soaks are optional. Antistaphylococcal antibiotics (e.g., penicillinase-resistant penicillin or cephalosporins) are usually given. Antibiotic coverage may need to be changed depending on the lack of clinical improvement and sensitivities of the cultured bacteria. The antibiotics should be used for an adequate time to allow for clinical improvement. Patients with osteomyelitis need 6 weeks of antibiotics. Home health care usually is not needed, except perhaps for dressing changes in the elderly or unreliable patient, with the patient who cannot use his or her other hand, or for the administration of home intravenous antibiotics. Inpatient treatment for intravenous antibiotics may be required in the diabetic or immunosup-

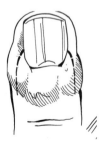

FIG. 7. Marsupialization of the eponychial fold for a chronic infection.

pressed patient, or the patient with a subungual abscess or osteomyelitis. Rehabilitation may be required in severe cases resulting in finger stiffness.

KEY POINTS

- Fingertip infections often can be treated in the office or emergency room.
- Complete débridement is imperative.
- Use culture-specific antibiotics.

HERPETIC WHITLOW

General Information

Herpes simplex infections of the digits are most commonly seen in people who occupationally expose their fingers to oral–tracheal secretions (e.g., dental personnel, anesthesiologists, and medical personnel in intensive and chronic care units). The incubation period between exposure and onset of symptoms is 2 to 14 days.

Diagnostic Criteria

The patient generally presents with a painful, clear vesicle(s) around the pad or nail. The size of the vesicles varies in size. Bacterial infection and skin ulceration may be present. Recurrence is common. A diagnosis is made by viral cultures, fluorescent antibody studies of the fluid from the vesicle, or a Tzanck smear.

Treatment

Symptomatic treatment is used. The infection is generally self-limiting. Antiviral medications (e.g., oral Acyclovir and ointment) may be used, especially in immunocompromised patients. Local dressings are applied to the lesions. Antibiotics are not used unless there is a secondary bacterial infection. Incision and drainage of the vesicles are contraindicated and may lead to viral encephalitis.

FLEXOR TENOSYNOVITIS

General Information

Suppurative flexor tenosynovitis is relatively common, accounting for approximately 10% of hand infections. These infections frequently occur following penetrating trauma but can also have a hematogenous origin. These injuries may seem trivial. The ring, middle, and index fingers are the most frequently involved digits. The most common offending organism is *Staphylococcus aureus.*

Diagnostic Criteria

Clinically, the patient complains of a painful, swollen, tender finger, that hurts worse with motion (Fig. 8). The pathognomonic signs of this condition (Kanavel's signs) include: (a) a semiflexed posture of the involved digit, (b) symmetrical swelling along the flexor tendon sheath, (c) tenderness and erythema along the flexor tendon sheath, and (d) severe pain on passive extension of the digit.

X-rays should be taken to rule out a foreign body in the involved digit.

Treatment

Nonoperative treatment may be indicated in the treatment of early suppurative flexor tenosynovitis with mild swelling and only 24 hours of symptoms. Treatment includes parenteral antibiotics, splint immobilization and elevation of the hand, and close serial observations.

Operative treatment is indicated in the treatment of moderate or severe symptoms, and in those patients who fail to respond to intravenous antibiotics. Treatment includes incisional drainage and irrigation. The surgical options include use of a proximal and distal incision along the flexor tendon sheath and use of an irrigation catheter (Fig. 9) or a volar Bruner incision. With use of an irrigation catheter, an incision is made along the proximal margin of the A1 pulley. A second incision is made and the distal margin of the flexor tendon sheath, either using a midlateral or volar incision. A no. 5 French feeding tube is placed from a proximal to distal direction. Irrigation solution is then placed through the feeding catheter initially in the operating room and postoperatively for 24 hours.

Infections involving the thumb or little finger can produce a horseshoe abscess if there is communication between the radial and ulnar bursas. Treatment should include débridement of all areas of infection.

The patient is placed on broad-spectrum antibiotics, including aerobic and anaerobic coverage. Antibiotic coverage may need to be changed, depending on the lack of clinical improvement and sensitivities of the cultured bacteria. The antibiotics should be used for an adequate time to allow for clinical improvement.

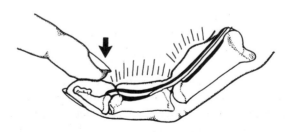

FIG. 8. Kanavel's cardinal signs for a flexor sheath infection.

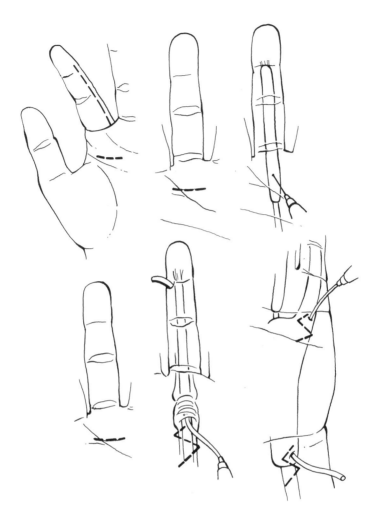

FIG. 9. Surgical incisions used to drain a flexor sheath infection.

DEEP SPACE INFECTIONS OF THE HAND

General Information

Deep space infections of the hand are relatively uncommon, accounting for approximately 2% of hand infections. The midpalmar and thenar spaces may be the site of abscesses following penetrating trauma. Midpalmar space infections can also result from rupture of a flexor tenosynovitis of the long, ring, or little finger or from distal palmar abscesses extending from the lumbrical canal. Thenar space infections can arise from a subcutaneous abscess of the thumb or index finger, tenosynovitis of the thumb or index finger, or as an extension of an infection of the radial bursa or midpalmar space.

The midpalmar space is that potential space that lies between the flexor tendons of the ulnar three digits (anteriorly) and the metacarpals and interosseous muscles (posteriorly). The thenar space is that potential space anterior to the adductor pollicis muscle, lying between the flexor tendons of the index finger and adductor muscle. The thenar and midpalmar spaces are separated by a fascial septum between the third metacarpal and palmar fascia (Chapter 2, Anatomy, Fig. 4).

Diagnostic Criteria

Clinically, the patient presents with pain in the affected area. The midpalmar space abscess presents with tenderness and swelling toward the ulnar side of the

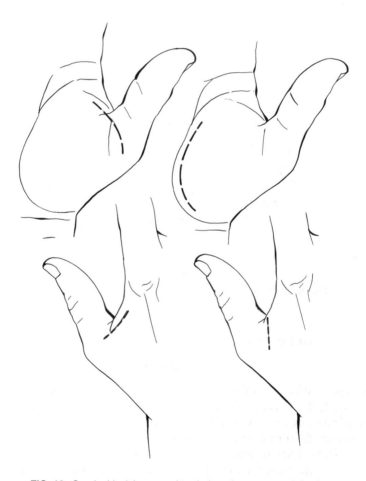

FIG. 10. Surgical incisions used to drain a thenar space infection.

midpalm. The thenar space abscess presents with similar findings in the thumb web space. The normal palmar concavity may be lost. The patient may present with more dorsal than palmar hand swelling, misleading the examiner of a possible palmar infection.

Treatment

Nonoperative treatment with antibiotics may be indicated in the treatment of early deep space infections, but in general these infections require operative débridement. The thenar space is débrided via a volar thenar incision or a dorsal first web space incision (Fig. 10).

The midpalmar space is débrided via a transverse palmar incision, a vertical palmar incision between third and fourth rays, or an oblique palmar incision (Fig. 11).

The patient is placed on broad-spectrum antibiotics, including aerobic and anaerobic coverage. Antibiotic coverage may need to be changed based on clinical improvement and sensitivities of the cultured bacteria. The antibiotics should be used for an adequate time to allow for clinical improvement.

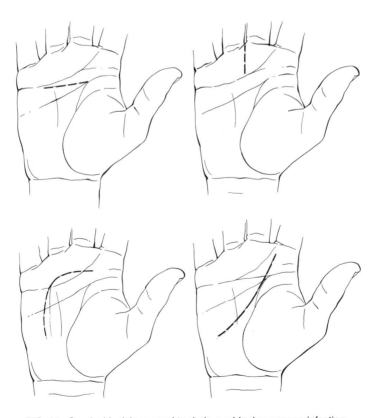

FIG. 11. Surgical incisions used to drain a midpalmar space infection.

ASCENDING LIMB INFECTIONS

General Information

Ascending limb infections pose a serious health risk and are frequently associated with some patients who have chronic diseases, senility, alcoholism, or drug abuse. Extensive trauma with devitalized trauma can also predispose the limb to an ascending limb infection. The causative organisms include *Clostridia, Streptococcus, Staphylococcus,* and various Gram-negative organisms.

Diagnostic Criteria

The patient usually presents with a swollen, painful, erythematous, enlarged arm. Cellulitis, lymphedema, and lymph node enlargement may be present. The condition may be life-threatening depending on the degree of infection. Subcutaneous crepitus may be present on physical examination. There is usually a significant elevation of the white blood cell count. X-rays may show the presence of subcutaneous air.

Treatment

Treatment incorporates immediate life support, including the placement of large-bore intravenous lines. All devitalized tissue should be débrided immediately. Multiple débridements may be necessary. The patient is placed on broad-spectrum antibiotics, including aerobic and anaerobic coverage. Antibiotic coverage may need to be changed depending on clinical improvement and sensitivities of the cultured bacteria.

SELECTED REFERENCES

Kanavel AB. Infections of the hand. A guide to the surgical treatment of acute and chronic and suppurative processes in the fingers, hand, and forearm, 7th ed. Lea and Febiger, Philadelphia, 1943.

Leddy JP. Infections of the upper extremity. J Hand Surg 1986;11A:294–297.

Linscheid RL, Dobyns JH. Common and uncommon infections of the hand. Orthop Clin North Am 1975;6:1063–1104.

Louis DS, Silva J Jr. Herpetic whitlow: herpetic infections of the digits. J Hand Surg 1979;4:90–94.

Neviaser RJ. Acute infections. In: Hotchkiss RN, Pederson WC, eds. Green's operative hand surgery, 4th ed. Churchill Livingstone, 1999, pp 1033–1047.

Neviaser RJ, Gunther GF. Tenosynovial infections of the hand. Part I: Acute pyogenic tenosynovitis of the hand. Instr Course Lect 1980;29:108–117.

22

Compartment Syndrome

GENERAL INFORMATION

An acute compartment syndrome occurs when the interstitial tissue pressure rises above the tissue perfusion pressure and causes a cycle of increasing edema and cellular necrosis. Acute compartment syndromes are subdivided into three groups that are related to the time of compartment pressurization: incipient, acute, and established. The end result of an untreated compartment syndrome can be hand and forearm contracture (Volkmann's ischemic contracture) or tissue loss. Compartment syndromes have a number of causes and can occur in both the hand and forearm.

DIAGNOSTIC CRITERIA

Maintaining a high index of suspicion for the development of the condition is critical to making the diagnosis. The diagnosis of compartment syndrome can be difficult, especially in cases where the interstitial tissue pressure is rising but does not yet meet the criteria for an established compartment syndrome. It may also be difficult in some clinical settings (e.g., after snakebite envenomation) where the symptoms of envenomation are similar to the symptoms of compartment syndrome.

These injuries are usually a result of a soft-tissue crushing injury (i.e., a roller injury). Cases of compartment syndrome have been reported following open and closed fractures, the application of circumferential casts, arterial laceration and repair (reperfusion), snakebite, external pressurization (drug addict lying on the arm for a prolonged period of time), medical anticoagulation, arterial puncture, hemophilic bleeding, and intraoperative limb positioning.

One of the earliest signs of compartment syndrome is pain out of proportion to the injury. Subsequently, patients describe loss of sensation and motor function. Sometimes, obtunded patients present for evaluation of limb swelling. In these cases an understanding of the conditions likely to be associated with compartment syndrome is valuable. On physical examination, the patient will have a tense swollen hand or forearm. Often the concave appearance of the palm

163

reverses and becomes convex. The earliest sign is "pain on passive stretch." Stretching muscles that pass through the compartment is painful for the patient. (For example, stretching the fingers into flexion is painful for patients with a volar forearm compartment syndrome. To test the intrinsic muscles of the hand for pain on passive stretch, place the metaphalangeal joint in extension and passively flex the interphalangeal joint.) Later, patients have abnormality on objective neurologic testing (loss of two-point discrimination and paralysis). Finally, patients lose skin coloration (pallor) and become pulseless. Patients can have a compartment syndrome with palpable pulses.

ASSESSMENT OF INTERSTITIAL TISSUE PRESSURE

The diagnosis is often made on the basis of the history and physical examination. Often, however, interstitial tissue pressure measurements are useful in confirming the diagnosis and effective treatment. Interstitial tissue pressures that are within 30 mm Hg of the mean arterial pressure or 20 mm Hg of the diastolic blood pressure are very suggestive of a compartment syndrome.

Interstitial tissue pressure measurements (ITPM) are reliable, objective observations that can be repeated during a period of observation. Do the following to measure the ITPM:

1. Assemble an "arterial line set up" and monitor.
2. Prepare the skin for puncture using Betadine solution.
3. Flush and zero the system.
4. Insert the 18-gauge catheter into the compartment (Fig. 1).
5. Read the pressure from the monitor.
6. Squeeze the compartment gently and observe the monitor for an increase in interstitial tissue pressure.
7. Remove the catheter and apply a Bandaid dressing.

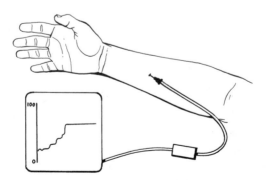

FIG. 1. Interstitial tissue pressure measurement set up.

To measure forearm compartments:

1. Volar forearm
2. Dorsal forearm
3. Mobile wad

To measure hand compartments:

1. Thenar muscles
2. Hypothenar muscles
3. Interossei muscles
   a. Between index and long metacarpals
   b. Between long ring and little metacarpals
4. Carpal canal pressure

The patient probably has an acute compartment syndrome if the ITPM is within 20 mm Hg of the diastolic blood pressure. If necessary, the ITPM should be measured every 2 to 3 hours to determine whether significant changes are occurring. Patients who are obtunded are excellent candidates for use of ITPM. Currently, no other imaging methods are widely used to make the diagnosis of compartment syndrome.

TREATMENT

The treatment for acute and established compartment syndrome is an emergency fasciotomy. Compartment syndrome is a major problem requiring urgent treatment. A fasciotomy is done in the operating room to decompress the forearm and hand. Specific incisions allow access to all of the compartments of the hand (Fig. 2). At the time of operation, the fascia is divided and the compartment

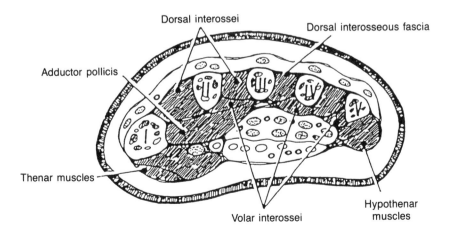

FIG. 2. Cross section showing the ten compartments of the hand.

muscle is inspected for evidence of necrosis. Devitalized tissue is resected and the wounds are left open. Serial débridements are done every 48 hours until the wound is stable. Closure is done using a delayed primary method of skin closure or split thickness skin grafting.

If the patient is medically anticoagulated or has a significant coagulation disorder, the coagulation properties should be corrected before undertaking fasciotomy whenever possible.

Early range of motion exercises should be begun as soon as possible to limit the formation of postoperative stiffness.

KEY POINTS

- A compartment syndrome can occur wherever muscles are enclosed in fascial envelopes.
- A high index of suspicion should be maintained for this condition when patients present with severe swelling.
- This diagnosis should be made using clinical examination.
- Measurement of the interstitial tissue pressure can obtain objective information.
- Patients with ongoing swelling and those who cannot communicate need serial ITPM to determine the need for fasciotomy.
- The outcome from early treatment is superior to the outcome from delayed treatment.

SELECTED REFERENCES

Whitesides TE, Haney TC, Harada H, Holmes HC, Morimoto K. A simple method for tissue pressure determination. Arch Surg 1975;110:1311–1313.[1]

---

[1]This article provides step-by-step instruction for the measurement of ITP.

23

Tumors

GANGLIONS

General Information

Ganglion cysts are the most common soft-tissue tumor of the hand. Ganglions are formed from modified synovial cells. The cyst is usually connected with an underlying joint or tendon sheath. A ganglion cyst usually occurs when there is a small tear in capsule allowing the synovial tissue to herniate out of its normal position.

Diagnostic Criteria

The patient presents with a soft-tissue mass. The mass may be painless or slightly painful. The mass tends to be nontender, semisoft, and will transilluminate. The mass can wax and wane as the cyst decompresses internally. The most common locations of the cyst are the dorsoradial wrist (originating from the dorsal scapholunate interosseous ligament) (Fig. 1), the volar radial wrist (originating from the volar radiocarpal joint) (Fig. 1), thumb carpometacarpal joint, or flexor carpi radialis tendon sheath), distal palm and proximal finger (a retinacular cyst originating from the tendon sheath between the A1 and A2 pulley) (Fig. 1), and dorsal distal finger (a mucous cyst originating from an arthritic distal interphalangeal joint) (Fig. 2).

Dorsal wrist ganglion cysts should be differentiated from dorsal extensor tenosynovitis and a dorsal carpometacarpal boss. Volar radial ganglion cysts should be differentiated from a radial artery aneurysm or traumatic pseudoaneurysm. An Allen's test to determine the patency of the ulnar artery should be performed prior to surgical excision. Retinacular cysts are small pea-sized masses that should be differentiated from a giant cell tumor, lipoma, or nerve tumor (e.g., neurilemmoma).

Treatment

Treatment options include observation, splinting, aspiration with or without steroid injection, or excision of the cyst. Aspiration of the cyst, with an 18-gauge

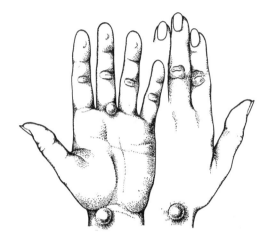

FIG. 1. Common sites for ganglion formation in the hand.

needle, may be indicated if the cyst is large or enlarging. Care should be taken in aspirating volar ganglion cysts owing to the presence of adjacent neurovascular structures. Injection of steroids and lidocaine may reduce the mass and symptoms for a varying amount of time. Recurrence following aspiration of the cyst is high (50% or more).

Definitive treatment includes removal of the ganglion and its origin. When excising a ganglion arising from the joint capsule or retinaculum, a small cuff of joint capsule or tendon sheath is also excised and left open. Excision of a mucous cyst from the distal interphalangeal joint also requires debridement of underlying joint osteophytes.

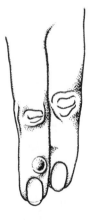

FIG. 2. A typical mucous cyst on the dorsum of a digit.

Operative excision of a cyst is associated with a significantly lower recurrence rate than aspiration and also allows for an accurate diagnosis.

GIANT CELL TUMORS OF TENDON SHEATH

General Information

Giant cell tumor (GCT) of tendon sheath is a benign soft-tissue tumor that is the second most common tumor of the hand. It has also been referred to as localized nodular synovitis, fibrous xanthoma, and pigmented villonodular tenosynovitis.

Diagnostic Criteria

The tumor is usually a slow growing, firm, nontender, and nodular mass. The tumor tends to occur along the volar aspect of the hand and fingers, although it can involve the dorsal aspect. It has a propensity for the radial three digits and the distal interphalangeal region. It may produce a sensory deficit secondary to digital nerve compression. In contrast to ganglions, the mass does not transilluminate.

X-rays reveal a soft tissue mass or occasionally erosion of underlying bone.

Treatment

Marginal excision is the usual treatment for a GCT. The risk of recurrence ranges from 5% to 50%. This high risk of recurrence may be secondary to the presence of satellite lesions or incomplete excision. Joint arthrodesis may be needed following tumor excision if extensive joint involvement or degenerative arthritis is noted. Malignant transformation of GCT is rare.

LIPOMAS

General Information

Lipomas are common benign fat tumors that occur in several locations in the hand. They are located subcutaneously, within muscles and the deep spaces of the hand.

Diagnostic Criteria

The tumors present as soft, nontender, slow-growing masses. They do not transilluminate. Symptoms of nerve compression may be present if the tumor is located near a peripheral nerve. Subcutaneous masses may be well demarcated.

X-rays reveal a soft-tissue mass. Magnetic resonance imaging reveals signal changes that are consistent with fat, which is usually similar to surrounding sub-cutaneous fat.

Treatment

Lipomas are generally excised. They tend to be well demarcated and are eas-ily dissected from surrounding tissue. Those tumors surrounding peripheral nerves should be carefully excised. An incisional biopsy is performed for those masses where the diagnosis is questionable.

GLOMUS TUMORS

General Information

Glomus tumors are formed from the vasculo-musculo-neuro "glomus" ele-ments of the nail bed that affect the regulation of blood flow. Proliferation of this angiomatous tissue may cause pressure on the nerve plexuses and exquisite pain.

Diagnostic Criteria

Glomus tumors are usually painful, subcutaneous nodules usually located in the subungual region of the digits. The patient presents with a severe, sharp, lan-cinating pain worsened by cold exposure or light touch. The physical examina-tion may be unremarkable in half of the patients. In some patients, a localized subungual bluish discoloration, with or without nail plate ridging, is present. Cold sensitivity may be provoked by immersion in an ice bath or spraying the digit with ethyl chloride.

A magnetic resonance image scan may show the lesion as a well-delineated bright spot on T2-weighted images.

Treatment

Symptomatic lesions are surgically excised. The nail plate is removed with lesions of the nail bed. The lesion is removed through a longitudinal incision made in the sterile matrix. Care is taken to remove the entire lesion and any other lesions present. There may be multiple lesions. Proximal lesions in the germinal matrix are removed through a dorsolateral skin incision. Small defects in the nail bed are closed primarily. Larger defects may be repaired with split-thickness nail bed grafts. Reexploration is considered in cases of incomplete pain relief or recurrence of symptoms.

ENCHONDROMAS

General Information

Enchondromas are benign cartilaginous lesions that are the most common benign hand bone tumors. Approximately 35% of all enchondromas arise in the hand and account for up to 90% of bone tumors in the hand. Most of these tumors occur in people between 10 and 40 years of age. The proximal phalanx is the most common site of involvement, followed by the metacarpal and middle phalanx.

Diagnostic Criteria

The patient may present with an asymptomatic lesion noted on x-rays taken of the hand for other reasons. They may also present with a pathologic fracture through the tumor. Radiographically, the tumor is noted to be a well-circum-scribed lytic lesion, which may be lobulated. Matrix calcification may also be seen. Soft-tissue extension is generally not noted.

Treatment

Small asymptomatic enchondromas may be observed. Large, symptomatic enchondromas generally requires biopsy, curettage, and usually bone grafting (autograft or allograft). Pathologic fractures may be treated acutely or following healing of the fracture. Recurrence of the tumor is treated with repeat curettage and grafting.

MALIGNANT SOFT-TISSUE TUMORS

General Information

Malignant soft-tissue tumors of the hand and forearm are uncommon. The more common cell types of soft-tissue sarcomas include epithelioid sarcoma, synovial cell sarcoma, and malignant fibrous histiocytoma.

Diagnostic Criteria

The patient usually presents with a mass that is generally painless and present for a long time, which may have recently started growing. Occasionally the mass may be painful. The mass may be misdiagnosed as an infection, ganglion, lipoma, or some other benign soft-tissue tumor. The patient should be assessed for the location and size of the tumor and the presence of regional lymph nodes.

Preoperative assessment should include x-rays, looking for soft-tissue calcification or bone involvement. Magnetic resonance imaging is used to assess the extent of the disease, including the size and depth of the lesion and the location of the tumor relative to surrounding bone, soft tissues, and neurovascular structures. Computed tomography (CT) is used if evidence exists of any bone involvement by the tumor.

Staging of the tumor, including a chest x-ray and CT of the chest and axilla, should be performed in the presence of a soft-tissue sarcoma.

Treatment

Symptomatic, enlarging soft-tissue tumors that are suspected of malignancy should be considered for biopsy. Small lesions may be treated with an excisional biopsy. A cuff of normal tissue should be removed at the time of surgery. Incisional biopsy is used for larger suspicious lesions. The biopsy should be performed with a longitudinal incision placed in a location allowing for limb-sparing surgery if indicated.

Soft-tissue sarcomas are graded based on the histologic grade, size of the tumor, and the presence of metastases. Surgical treatment should include removal of the tumor with a cuff of normal surrounding tissue. The use of adjunctive treatment (brachytherapy, external beam radiation, and chemotherapy) either preoperatively or postoperatively depends on the tumor type and size, the presence of metastases, and whether adequate excision of the tumor is possible. An amputation is considered for those tumors in which adequate resection is not possible or tumors that have been inadequately excised and cannot be adequately reexcised. The treatment of these tumors requires close collaboration among the surgeon, pathologist, oncologist, radiologist, and radiation oncologist.

MALIGNANT BONE TUMORS

General Information

Malignant bone tumors of the hand and forearm are uncommon. The more common types include chondrosarcoma, osteogenic sarcoma, Ewing's sarcoma, and metastatic tumors. Chondrosarcoma is the most common primary malignant bone tumor that occurs in the hand. The tumor may arise primarily or may develop in a preexistent benign tumor (e.g., enchondroma, osteochondroma). The lesion most commonly occurs in patients over the age of 60. The proximal phalanges and metacarpals are most commonly affected. Osteogenic and Ewing's sarcomas and metastatic tumors are rarely seen in the hand. Osteogenic sarcomas occur in older patients (fourth to sixth decade of life), whereas Ewing's sarcoma occurs in younger patients (first to second decade of life). These tumors occur most commonly in the metacarpals or phalanges. Metastatic tumors occur as, preterminal events. They often are a part of a widespread dissemination of a primary carcinoma and occur most frequently in the distal phalanx or other phalanges.

Diagnostic Criteria

The clinical presentation varies with the tumor type. Some patients present with a slow-growing, firm mass (chondrosarcoma) versus a rapidly enlarging mass (osteogenic sarcoma), or with symptoms resembling an infection (Ewing's sarcoma). Swelling, erythema, and systemic illness may be present (Ewing's sarcoma).

Preoperative assessment should include radiographs. Patients with chondrosarcomas usually present with x-rays that demonstrate stippled calcification, cortical expansion, but can have cortical perforation, and possible soft-tissue extension of the tumor. Osteogenic sarcomas have an expansile, sclerotic lesion with malignant new bone formation or a lytic or mixed pattern with bone destruction and soft-tissue mass. Ewing's sarcoma has a large lytic, destructive extensile lesion.

Computed tomography is used to determine the degree of cortical involvement and tumor penetration. Magnetic resonance imaging is used to assess the extent of the tumor within the medullary canal and in the surrounding soft tissue if cortical penetration has occurred. Staging of the patient should include a chest x-ray and CT of the chest to rule out metastases.

Treatment

Patients with a suspected malignant bone tumor should be considered for a biopsy and intraoperative cultures. The biopsy should be performed with a longitudinal incision placed in a location allowing for limb-sparing surgery if indicated. The resection of malignant bone tumors of the hand generally requires some form of en bloc resection of the lesion, ray resection, or amputation. Adjuvant radiation or chemotherapy may be indicated depending on tumor type. The primary aim in treating metastatic tumors is to relieve pain and preserve function. Treatment may include ray resection or amputation, curettage and packing with methylmethacrylate, and radiation therapy.

24

Arthritis

OSTEOARTHRITIS

General Information

In degenerative arthritis or osteoarthritis of the hand, the most commonly involved joints are the distal interphalangeal joints (DIPJ), proximal interphalangeal joints (PIPJ), and thumb carpometacarpal (CMC) joint. The metacarpophalangeal joints (MCPJ) are rarely involved. Marginal osteophytes, producing enlargement of the DIPJ and PIPJ, are known as Heberden's and Bouchard's nodes, respectively (Fig. 1).

ARTHRITIS OF THE BASILAR JOINT OF THE THUMB

General Information

Pain and loss of function may result from primary osteoarthritis, posttraumatic arthritis, or rheumatoid arthritis of the carpometacarpal joint of the thumb. Arthritis causes a reduction of pinch and grip strength and necessitates adaptive movements to avoid painful motion of this joint. The joint may narrow, stiffen, and/or subluxate. A resultant adduction deformity of the thumb metacarpal may lead to a secondary hyperextension deformity or other disabling instabilities of the thumb metacarpophalangeal joint. The osteoarthritis may have a genetic basis and be associated with osteoarthritis of other joints. Posttraumatic arthritis may develop from fractures of dislocations of the base of the first metacarpal that result in incongruity of subluxation of the joint. In rheumatoid disease, joint damage results from synovial disease. Osteoarthritis is more common over the age of 40 and approximately three times more common in women than men. Carpal tunnel syndrome occurs with increased frequency in patients with thumb basilar joint arthritis.

Diagnostic Criteria

Clinically, the patient presents with pain with use of the thumb. Swelling or deformity of the basilar joint may be present. There may be a history of a previ-

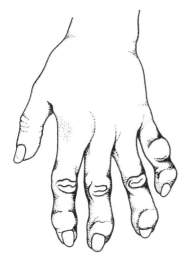

FIG. 1. Osteoarthritis of the hand.

ous joint injury or rheumatoid arthritis. On physical examination, tenderness and/or dorsoradial subluxation of the thumb carpometacarpal joint is noted. The axial compression-adduction test (Fig. 2) is done by manipulating the thumb with axial compression and adduction. Pain, joint instability, and crepitus are noted at the arthritic carpometacarpal joint.

The axial compression and rotation or grind test (Fig. 3) is performed by compressing and rotating the proximal phalanx and metacarpal of the thumb on the trapezium. Pain is noted at the CMC joint.

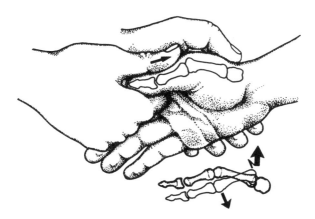

FIG. 2. Axial compression-adduction test of the thumb carpometacarpal joint.

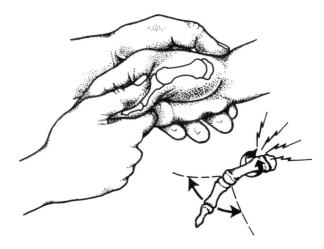

FIG. 3. Axial compression and rotation or grind test of the thumb carpometacarpal joint.

The relocation test (Fig. 4) is done by placing pressure on the base of a dorsally and radially subluxed thumb metacarpal. Placing pressure in a volar and ulnar direction reduces the CMC joint. Pain is noted at the CMC joint.

The first web space may be contracted. The thumb metacarpophalangeal joint may show a secondary hyperextension deformity or other instability pattern. Pinch and grip strength is frequently reduced. Thenar atrophy may be seen in advanced cases. De Quervain's tenosynovitis should be ruled out as the cause of thumb pain.

Radiographs of the thumb should include all the joints of the thumb, including the carpometacarpal and scaphotrapeziotrapezoid joint. On rare occasion, tomograms, or computed tomographic scanning (CT scan) may be used to better demonstrate involvement of the scaphotrapeziotrapezoid joint.

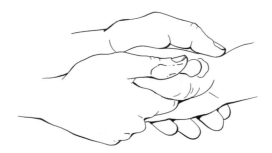

FIG. 4. Relocation test of the thumb carpometacarpal joint.

Treatment

Nonoperative treatment is indicated in those patients with mild symptoms, those who have had no previous treatment, or those who have a medical contraindication for surgery. Nonoperative options include activity modification, a thumb spica splint, nonsteroidal antiinflammatory drugs, and steroid injections. Those patients with rheumatoid arthritis may benefit from treatment of their underlying illness. Therapeutic modalities may include heat, whirlpool, and other similar modalities. Job and activity of daily activities modification, adaptive devices, and strengthening exercises may be beneficial.

Surgery is indicated to treat progressive symptoms of disabling pain, limitation of motion, and adduction contracture of the thumb basilar joint, in patients who have failed nonoperative treatment. Surgical treatment options vary widely and include total or partial trapezium excision with soft-tissue interposition arthroplasty; partial or complete trapezium excision with oblique ligament reconstruction; silicone implant trapezium replacement arthroplasty; cemented or uncemented total joint arthroplasty; and arthrodesis of the carpometacarpal joint.

Postoperative rehabilitation includes elevation of the hand with exercise of the fingers, elbow, and shoulder. Thumb and wrist splinting/casting is performed up to 8 weeks postoperatively. Range of motion exercises, strengthening exercises, patient education for activities of daily living, and job modification are performed. Adaptive devices may be needed.

INFLAMMATORY ARTHRITIS

General Information

In contrast to degenerative or osteoarthritis, which affects the hyaline cartilage in diarthrodial joints, inflammatory arthritis is a systemic disorder. In addition to joint problems, these patients frequently present with systemic symptoms such as skin rashes and ulcers, organ (cardiac, pulmonary, renal, gastrointestinal) dysfunction, hematologic disorders, and Raynaud's phenomenon. The more common of these disorders include rheumatoid arthritis, systemic lupus erythematosus, psoriatic arthritis, and scleroderma.

Rheumatoid arthritis is a systemic condition affecting synovial tissue. The deformities of the hand resulting from rheumatoid arthritis are secondary to hypertrophied synovial tissues. The deformities seen in rheumatoid arthritis include joint destruction, tendon ruptures, and loss of the normal configuration of the hand because of loss of the normal muscle, tendon, and ligament soft-tissue balances in the hand.

Diagnostic Criteria

The patient presents with a stiff wrist and fingers. The fingers may be swollen and painful. The metacarpophalangeal (MCP) and proximal interphalangeal

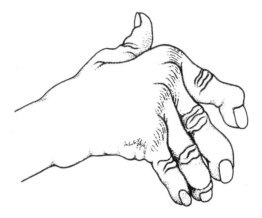

FIG. 5. Rheumatoid arthritis of the hand with ulnar drift deformity of the digits.

(PIP) joints are the most commonly involved. Morning stiffness and pain are common. With disease progression, joint deformity with radial deviation of the wrist and ulnar drift deformities of the digits (Fig. 5) are common.

Swan neck (Fig. 6) and boutonniere (Fig. 7) deformities are common. Other problems that may be present include joint synovitis or arthritis, flexor and extensor tenosynovitis or ruptures, carpal tunnel syndrome, and trigger fingers.

Treatment

There are generally five types of surgery used to treat the rheumatoid hand: joint synovectomy, tenosynovectomy, tendon surgery (repair or reconstruction), arthroplasty, or arthrodesis. The indications for surgery vary from one patient to another. The general indications for surgical intervention include providing pain relief, minimizing deformity, and improving function and appearance.

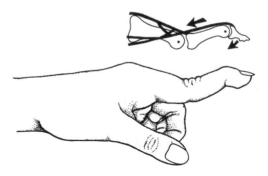

FIG. 6. Swan neck deformity of the finger with dorsal subluxation of the lateral bands.

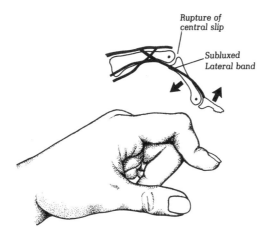

Rupture of
central slip

Subluxed
Lateral band

FIG. 7. Boutonniere deformity of the finger with rupture of the central slip and volar subluxation of the lateral bands.

Synovectomy is indicated in those patients with mild disease controlled with medical treatment but who have persistent joint synovitis without significant joint arthritis. Tenosynovectomy is indicated in patients with persistent tenosynovitis to prevent tendon ruptures or during tendon reconstruction. Tendon surgery includes the repair of ruptured tendons (direct repair, tendon grafts, tendon transfers) and tendon realignment procedures. Joint arthroplasty or arthrodesis is usually indicated for patients with painful arthritis of the wrist and finger joints.

SELECTED REFERENCES

Berger RA, Beckenbaugh RD, Linscheid RL. Arthroplasty in the hand and wrist. In:
Green DP, Hotchkiss RN, Pederson WC, eds. Green's operative hand surgery, Churchill-Livingstone, Philadelphia, 1999, pp. 147–191.
Burton RI, Pelligrini VD. Surgical management of basal joint arthritis of the thumb. Pt II.
Ligament reconstruction with tendon interposition arthroplasty. J Hand Surg 1986;11A:324–332.
Feldon P, Terrono AL, Nalebuff EA, Millender LH. Rheumatoid arthritis and other connective tissue diseases. In: Green DP, Hotchkiss RN, Pederson WC, eds. Green's operative hand surgery, Churchill-Livingstone, Philadelphia, 1999, pp 1651–1739.
Millender LH, Nalebuff EA. Degenerative arthritis I. Hand Clin 1987;3:325–453.
Millender LH, Nalebuff EA. Degenerative arthritis II. Hand Clin 1987;3:455–627.
Millender LH, Nalebuff EA. Reconstructive surgery in the rheumatoid hand. Orthop Clin North Am 1975;6:709–732.

25

Tendonitis of the Wrist and Hand

GENERAL INFORMATION

Tendonitis of the hand and wrist is a common upper extremity disorder. Tendonitis should not be used as a "waste basket" term to diagnose generalized wrist and hand pain, but should refer to a specific anatomic site. Three common tendon afflictions are tenosynovitis, tenovaginitis, and tendinosis. Any tendon or group of tendons that have a synovial lining can become inflamed (tenosynovitis). A tendon can be constricted by a tight covering or sheath (tenovaginitis). A tendon origin or insertion can become diseased or degenerated secondary to age, poor blood supply, friction, or overuse (tendinosis). The three conditions may occur as independent entities or in combination.

DE QUERVAIN'S TENDONITIS

De Quervain's tendonitis refers to involvement of the tendons of the first dorsal compartment (abductor pollicis longus [APL] and the extensor pollicis brevis [EPB] tendons). Within the compartment, the APL has multiple tendinous slips and is often separated from the EPB by a septum. De Quervain's tendonitis is associated with repetitive tasks involving the thumb and wrist, as well as with pregnancy and childcare. Patients have tenderness over the first dorsal compartment and pain during a Finkelstein's test (asking the patient to fully flex the thumb and passively move the wrist into ulnar deviation). This maneuver is positive if it reproduces the patient's discomfort. Typically, active thumb abduction and extension against resistance is painful. The differential diagnosis for radial-sided wrist pain includes thumb carpometacarpal or scaphotrapezoid joint arthritis, scaphoid fracture or nonunion, radiocarpal arthritis, radial styloid fracture, and radial sensory neuritis (Wartenberg's syndrome). An x-ray of the wrist should be obtained if there is any question about the diagnosis.

TABLE 1. *Principles of tendon sheath injection*

3-mL syringe with 25-gauge needle
Solution preparation ($\frac{1}{2}$ cc 1*% plain lidocaine and $\frac{1}{2}$ cc corticosteroid)
Sterile preparation of site
Introduce solution within the sheath
Inject and observe filling within the sheath, avoid intratendinous injection
Apply Bandaid

Treatment

Nonsurgical treatment of De Quervain's tendonitis includes rest, antiinflammatory medication, stretching exercises, and corticosteroid injections. A forearm-based thumb spica splint immobilizes the APL and EPB tendons. Corticosteroid injection is used to deliver a bolus of antiinflammatory medication to the site of inflammation (Table 1). A steroid preparation that is partially or totally water-soluble is recommended to limit the local effects of steroid deposition; subcutaneous fat atrophy, and cutaneous depigmentation. In addition, passing the needle to the radius and pulling back slightly ensures the injection is deep within the sheath (Fig. 1). Persistent pain that is refractory to nonsurgical treatment warrants surgical release of the extensor compartment by incising the overlying retinaculum.

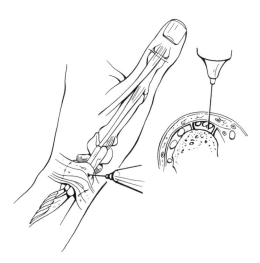

FIG. 1. Intracompartmental injection for De Quervain's tendonitis is placed just proximal to the radial styloid. Tendons are palpated by having patient perform a resisted thumb abduction maneuver and site is marked. The 25-gauge needle is placed through the tendon to bone, and then pulled back slightly. The medication injection then proceeds without much resistance.

OTHER AREAS OF TENDONITIS

Tendonitis can also occur in any of the other dorsal compartments and treatment is similar to De Quervain's. Second compartment tendonitis is called intersection syndrome and occurs where the wrist extensors pass under the first compartment muscles. Third compartment tendonitis affects the extensor pollicis longus tendon as it wraps around Lister's tubercle and is common after distal radius fractures. Persistent inflammation can result in an attritional extensor pollicis longus tendon rupture. Sixth compartment tendonitis affects the extensor carpi ulnaris tendon and may be related to underlying distal radioulnar joint pathology (e.g., instability or triangular fibrocartilage tear).

The palmar aspect of the wrist is less commonly affected by tendonitis. The flexor carpi radialis tendon resides within a separate fibroosseous compartment adjacent to the carpal tunnel. Tenosynovitis affecting the flexor carpi radialis tendon can be particularly recalcitrant to nonoperative measures.

TRIGGER DIGITS (FINGERS AND THUMBS)

Flexor tendons travel through a digital sheath between the metacarpophalangeal (MCP) and distal interphalangeal (DIP) joints. A discrepancy between the diameter of the tendons and the amount of sheath opening causes triggering. Patients initially complain of pain over the palmar aspect of the MCP joint. Later they will have triggering of the tendons on entrance into the sheath. Pain is often perceived at the proximal interphalangeal (PIP) joint of the finger or the inter-

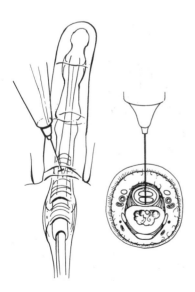

FIG. 2. Trigger digit injection for finger is placed 90 degrees to flexor sheath at level of proximal finger flexor crease. (For thumb, place 1 cm proximal to interphalangeal flexion crease.) The 25-gauge needle is placed in the midline, through the flexor tendon(s) to the bone. The needle is pulled back slightly to the point where the medication flows smoothly.

phalangeal (IP) joint of the thumb. Tenderness to palpation over the first annular pulley is common. Over time, locking of the finger in flexion can occur, as the tendon is unable to pass into the sheath. Passive manipulation of the digit into extension is required to alleviate the pain. Continued locking can result in a PIP joint flexion contracture. Trigger digits are common in patients with diabetes mellitus.

Treatment

Nonsurgical treatment includes rest and corticosteroid injection. Splinting of the PIP joints of the fingers or interphalangeal joint of the thumb in extension averts triggering and prevents continued irritation of the tendon(s). Corticosteroid injection into the flexor sheath often provides relief of mild to moderate triggering. The solution should be placed within the sheath; an intratendinous injection must be avoided (Fig. 2). Surgery is required for persistent symptoms and involves release of the first annular pulley.

ELBOW TENDINOSIS

Lateral (tennis elbow) epicondylitis is a result of degeneration and microtears of the extensor carpi radialis brevis origin (Fig. 3). Activities that emphasize wrist extension (e.g., tennis backhand, hammering) are associated with lateral epicondylitis. The pain is localized just anterior to the lateral epicondyle and elicited by forceful wrist extension. The pain is typically worse with the elbow extended since it stretches the extensor origin. The differential diagnosis includes radial tunnel syndrome and joint problems (e.g., instability or arthritis).

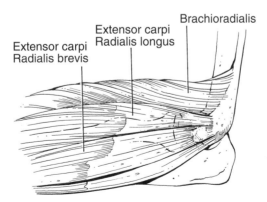

FIG. 3. Lateral epicondylitis. Degenerative lesion at the origin of the extensor carpi radialis brevis, located anterior (not directly lateral) on the lateral epicondyle.

Treatment

The mainstay of treatment is nonsurgical management, which is effective in 80% to 90% of individuals. Activity modification, therapeutic modalities (i.e., stretching, heat), and use of a counterforce brace are employed. A corticosteroid injection near the origin of the extensor carpi radialis brevis origin is useful.

MEDIAL EPICONDYLITIS

Medial epicondylitis (golfer's elbow) is less common. The tendinosis is at the origin of the flexor/pronator muscle group (Fig. 4). Pain is referred to the flexor pronator origin with resisted wrist flexion and pronation and not with resisted extension of the fingers or wrist.

Treatment

Treatment is similar to lateral epicondylitis. The differential diagnosis is cubital tunnel (entrapment of the ulnar nerve at the elbow) or elbow joint/ligament pathology.

KEY POINTS

- Tendonitis is a diagnosis that should refer to a specific tendon or group of tendons.
- The diagnosis is confirmed by maneuvers that cause pain isolated to the tendon(s) by stretching or use against resistance.
- Nonsurgical treatment consists of rest, splinting, antiinflammatory medication, stretching exercises, and corticosteroid injections.

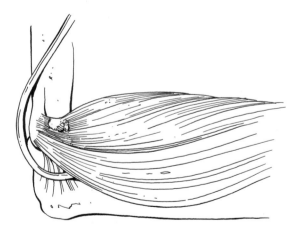

FIG. 4. Medial epicondylitis. The figure shows a degenerative lesion at the origin of the flexor pronator origin on anterior aspect of the medial epicondyle. Note proximity to the ulnar nerve.

SELECTED REFERENCES

Bennett JB. Lateral and medial epicondylitis. Hand Clin 1994,10:157–163.

Rhoades CE, Gelberman RH, Manjarris JF. Stenosing tenosynovitis of the fingers and thumb. Results of a prospective trial of steroid injection and splinting. Clin Orthop 1984;190:236–238.

Weiss AP, Akelman E, Tabatabai M. Treatment of De Quervain's disease. J Hand Surg (Am) 1994;19:595–597.

Witt J, Pess G, Gelberman RH. Treatment of De Quervain tenosynovitis: a prospective study of the results of infection of steroids and immobilization in a splint. Bone Joint Surg 1991;73(2)219–221.

26

Burns

GENERAL INFORMATION

Thermal burns to the hand occur as a result of energy dissipated from flame, liquid, or gas. Chemical burns arise from direct contact with acidic or extremely alkaline substances. Electrical burns result from the energy dissipated when an electrical current passes through tissue. These injuries commonly occur in occupational situations.

DIAGNOSTIC CRITERIA

It is extremely important to determine the method of burning. The duration of exposure and temperature of the flame should be determined for thermal burns. The nature of the agent must be identified for chemical burns. Current density, duration of contact, the pathway through the body, and the patient's premorbid medical status should all be identified before treatment is initiated for electrical burns.

Thermal Burns

Burns with skin destruction are referred to as either partial-thickness or full-thickness, depending on the depth of skin and subcutaneous destruction (Fig. 1). Partial-thickness burns may be characterized by erythema, tender skin, or blistering. The skin is red, moist, and blanches with pressure. Burns causing partial-thickness injury are painful. Full-thickness burns may leave the skin dry, hard, white, or even charred. Full-thickness burns destroy the sensory nerve fibers and often are not painful. The size of the injured area of skin should be measured.

Chemical Burns

The skin is often blotchy with blisters in chemical burns. Hydrofluoric acid is a common ingredient in rust removers and is widely used in the glass etching industry. Contact with the skin can cause particularly painful lesions. Sulfuric

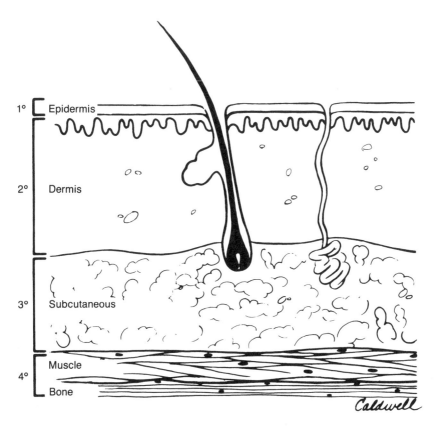

FIG. 1. Skin depth assessment.

acid is found in car batteries and is an occupational hazard for mechanics. Hydrochloric acid is used in toilet and pool-cleaning solvents. Sodium hypochlorite is found in bleach and other household solvents.

Electrical Burns

Patients with electrical burns often present with red and swollen skin. Although skin injury may occur at either entry or exit, charring is frequently seen where the current exits the body. The examiner should carefully look for "arc wounds," where the current jumps from one skin surface to another, such as in the axilla. Necrotic tissue may exist anywhere between the entrance and exit regions of the current. Electrical injuries may be classified as either low-tension (<1,000 V) or high-tension (>1,000 V). Electrical injuries are uncommon when the current is less than 500 V.

TREATMENT

Superficial thermal burns can be treated with medicated lotions, such as aloe vera, ice, or moist towels. Mild analgesics and nonsteroidal antiinflammatory drugs (NSAIDs) may be helpful for pain. Full recovery can be anticipated in 5 to 7 days. More advanced partial-thickness burns and some full-thickness thermal burns are treated with silver sulfadiazine, silver nitrate, or mafenide acetate creams, healing by secondary intention. Analgesics and NSAIDs may also be used for electrical burns.

The treating physician must first focus on the "ABCs" of evaluation and resuscitation for extensive burns. Extensive thermal burns can be associated with large fluid and nutrient leakage as a result of the loss of skin integrity. Severe electrical burns can produce cardiac arrhythmias, seizures, and severe muscle and nerve necrosis. Renal failure may result from myoglobinuria produced from muscle necrosis. Full-thickness skin loss greater than 3 cm in diameter generally requires prompt coverage, not only for functional purposes but also for retention of fluids and nutrients. Meshed split-thickness skin grafts are used to cover areas of healthy granulation tissue. Occasionally, pedicle or free flaps are used for areas of exposed tendon or bone.

Compartment syndrome must be considered for severe burns with tissue necrosis or burns associated with tissue necrosis. Compartment pressures should be measured and compartment releases and escharotomies performed when necessary. In general, large thermal burns and severe electrical burns with full-thickness damage require urgent escharotomy or débridement. Repeat operative débridements will likely be necessary to remove devitalized skin, subcutaneous tissue, and muscle tissue. Decompression of peripheral nerves is also usually necessary. The hand should be positioned in the "safe position" for burns directly involving the hand and digits. Patients with hand burns often need prolonged periods of intensive hand rehabilitation.

One should remove all clothing in contact with the chemical and irrigate the burned area with large volumes of water for 20 minutes or longer for treatment of chemical burns. Acid burns may be treated with diluted sodium bicarbonate. Alkaline burns can be neutralized with dilute acetic acid. Phenol (carbolic acid) burns can be treated with ethyl alcohol. Hydrofluoric acid burns tend to spread beneath the skin, becoming extremely painful. Hydrofluoric acid burns can be treated with subcutaneous injections of 10% calcium gluconate and topical 2.5% calcium gluconate gel and are applied until pain is relieved. Formal skin and soft-tissue débridement including nail removal may be necessary.

COLD INJURY

As in burns, injury from exposure to cold is directly related to the temperature and length of exposure. The severity of the injury is directly affected by the following factors: wetness, dependency, vasospasm, open wounds, body position, and constrictive clothing. All too often, the patient may not realize that cold injury is occurring. The initial symptoms of cold injury are itching or a sensation of burning, also referred to as "chilblains." These symptoms progress to numbness and extreme coldness of the affected area as frostbite occurs. Fluid vesicles, ulcers, or incomplete skin and dermal loss may occur with the development of partial-thickness cold injury. Cold injury may progress to full-thickness skin and dermal loss requiring skin or free-tissue coverage. Deep injury to muscle, tendon, or bone can also occur.

The initial treatment for cold injury is cessation of exposure to the source of cold followed by the removal of all cold and wet clothing. Gentle rewarming of the extremity is then performed using water at the temperature of 40 to 42°C. The hand and digits are then dressed and splinted, using the principles previously discussed. The rewarming period may be very painful and analgesics may be required. Permanent cold sensitivity may result, and extensive hand therapy may be required. Although surgical treatment is occasionally necessary to remove devitalized tissue, it is best done after all soft-tissue changes have occurred.

SELECTED REFERENCES

Danielson JR, Capelli-Schellpfeffer M, Lee RC. Upper extremity electrical injury. Hand Clin 2000;16: 225–233.
Reilly DA, Garner WL. Management of chemical injuries to the upper extremity. Hand Clin 2000;16: 215–223.
Tredget EE. Management of the acutely burned upper extremity. Hand Clin 2000;16:187–203.

27

High-Pressure Injection Injuries

GENERAL INFORMATION

High-pressure injection injuries (HPII) occur when patients sustain an injury from a high-pressure injection tool. Usually, the material that is injected is an organic solvent that causes significant tissue death.

DIAGNOSTIC CONSIDERATIONS

History

Patients usually present for evaluation of finger or hand injuries that were sustained while using a high-pressure tool for painting, lubrication or doing maintenance on diesel fuel injectors. Injury usually occurs when the operator wipes a blocked nozzle or tries to steady the gun with his or her free (nondominant) hand. The pain may be mild if it has been a short time since the injury. Initial local symptoms include pain, swelling, and numbness. Often, the pain is severe after a few hours and usually tracks along the line of injection (Fig. 1). Ask the patient what material was used in the device at the time of injection. The four most common substances injected are grease, paint, pain solvent, and diesel fuel. Injection injuries have been reported with water, air, hydraulic fuel, and cement. Patients should be asked about hand dominance and the last time of tetanus immunization.

Physical Examination

Only a small site of the injection may be seen early in the course of this condition. A careful assessment should be made of the location of the injection and the route of the injected material. Over time, a significant increase in edema is common. The increase in edema may be associated with impaired arterial inflow and venous drainage (compartment syndrome) (Chapter 22, Compartment Syn-

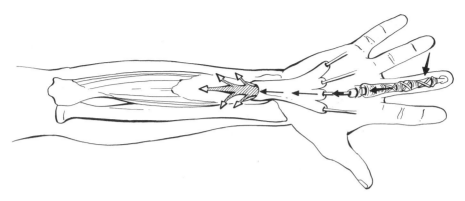

FIG. 1. Palmar wounds at high pressure may spread into the proximal forearm.

drome, Fig. 1). The early appearance of these wounds is seemingly innocuous. The material can be injected from the fingertip to the elbow if a synovial space has been opened. If the material is injected into the subcutaneous space, it can be expected to spread locally, often down the path of the digital nerves and arteries. The entire arm should be examined for local tenderness along a musculo-tendinous unit that indicates the path of injection.

After several months or years, skin breakdown over the oleogranulomas can lead to the formation of ulcers and draining sinuses. These sinuses can become secondarily infected.

X-rays may be helpful in demonstrating the path of the injected material in the finger, hand, and forearm.

TREATMENT

High-pressure injection injuries are major problems requiring urgent treatment. Almost always, patients with injection injuries need early operative débridement to remove the injected material. Injected materials that are organic solvents cause progressive tissue death; these should be removed as soon as possible. The main surgical principles are decompression and débridement. Necrotic tissue should be resected at the time of surgery. Serial débridements are done every 48 hours until the wound improves. Skin closure can be complex in these cases. Antimicrobial therapy should include tetanus prophylaxis and broad-spectrum antibiotics (first-generation cephalosporin and aminoglycoside).

The hand should be splinted in the "safe position." Following débridement, early range of motion exercises should be instituted to limit the formation of finger and hand stiffness.

KEY POINTS

- Grease guns can generate a nozzle pressure of up to 10,000 pounds per square inch (similar to the muzzle velocity of a rifle).
- The criteria for diagnosis are a history of an injury from a high-pressure injection tool, an identifiable site of injection, and pain along the path of the injected material.
- Skin contact with the nozzle is not required to produce serious injury.
- The pattern of injury is determined by
  —Location of injection.
  —Resistance of structures encountered.
  —Anatomy of the compartment.
  —Viscosity of the material injected.
  —Pressure of injection.
  —Volume of material injected.

SELECTED REFERENCES

Trawick RH, Seiler JG, Kasdan ML. High pressure injection injuries to the hand. Occup Disord 1998; 373–379.

28

Bites

HUMAN BITES

General Information

Human bites commonly occur on the hand following fights (fight bite) (Fig. 1). These wounds are often complicated by bacteriologic infection because of the complex flora of the human mouth.

Diagnostic Criteria

Physical Examination

The bites are usually located over the extensor surface of the hand in the vicinity of the metacarpophalangeal joints. One should inspect the area of the bite for evidence of infection and palpate the adjacent joints to look for evidence of septic arthritis.

Other Assessment

Patients with evidence of infection should have a white blood count with a differential. Radiographs should be done if there is a concern for fracture, septic arthritis, or osteomyelitis.

Treatment

All wounds should be explored to determine the depth of the bite. The extensor tendon should be inspected. During the exploration, specific inspection of the joint capsule should be done to determine if the bite extends to the joint space. The finger should be examined in both flexion and extension.

Superficial wounds can be treated with irrigation and débridement. Tetanus immunization should be updated whenever appropriate. Usually these wounds are treated with twice daily dressing changes until the wounds heal by secondary

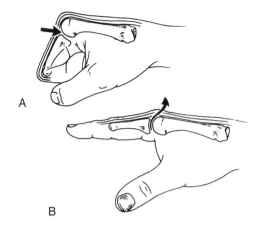

A

B

FIG. 1. A: A tooth penetrates the fully flexed metacarpophalangeal joint of a closed fist. **B:** As the digit is extended, the inoculum is trapped because the path of entrance is now closed.

intention. Patients should be instructed in range of motion exercises for the hand to limit the occurrence of stiffness.

Deep wounds and wounds with joint space involvement should be treated by extending the wound and thoroughly irrigating the joint and tendon space. The wounds should be packed open and the patient should be instructed in local care.

Often these patients need intravenous antibiotics. Patients with established bone and joint infection need early referral to a hand specialist.

KEY POINTS

- *Staphylococcus aureus* is the most common organism causing hand infections after human bite. *Eikenella corrodens* can also cause infection following human bite.
- One should carefully inspect the wound to evaluate for joint space penetration or early septic arthritis. Satisfactory débridement is crucial to obtaining a good outcome.
- Initial antibiotic therapy usually requires both a first-generation cephalosporin and penicillin. Culture results give the physician the opportunity to use specific antibiotics.

CAT AND DOG BITES

General Information

Cat and dog bites are the most common bites seen for emergency evaluation. Untreated, these bites are commonly complicated by infection, often by *alpha Streptococcus, Staphylococcus aureus,* and *Pasteurella multocida.*

Diagnostic Criteria

History

Most often patients are bitten or scratched on the hand when attempting to handle the animal. It is important to determine whether the bite was provoked in some way. If the bite was not provoked, then rabies prophylaxis should be considered. These bites are often painful and associated with the early onset of infection.

Physical Examination

The physical examination should include recording the patient's temperature, observing the bites for location and number; careful assessment for local tenderness, erythema, subcutaneous abscess, and deep infection; palpation of the arm for evidence of abscess, ascending infection, and tender proximal adenopathy.

Other Assessment

Patients who have developed a significant infection or abscess require a complete blood count.

Treatment

Usually the wounds are small puncture sites that may need to be opened with an incision to allow thorough inspection of the bite and débridement of devitalized tissue. Obtain cultures of any suspicious fluid. Usually the wound should be left open to granulate. When indicated, update the tetanus status. The patient should be instructed to perform twice-daily dressing changes and issued a prescription for oral antibiotics (usually Augmentin).

Aftercare

Patients should be followed carefully to look for evidence of bite site infection. Patients should be instructed in range of motion exercises and twice-daily dressing changes. Some patients may benefit from more intensive local wound care methods (whirlpool treatments) and organized occupational therapy

KEY POINTS

- Rabies has been reported after domestic cat bite. If the animal cannot be observed, the local health department should be consulted for advice on rabies prophylaxis. One should always determine the rabies immunization status of the biting animal.

- The deep spaces of the hand are often inoculated because of the configuration of the animal's tooth.
- These infections are usually caused by the normal flora of the animal's mouth.
- Patients who present with an established hand abscess usually need intravenous antibiotics, serial débridement, and intensive occupational therapy.

SELECTED REFERENCE

Goldstein EJ. Bite wounds and infection. Clin Infect Dis 1992;14:633–638.

OTHER "WILD ANIMAL" BITES

Unusual wild animal bites (raccoons, skunks, foxes, bats, and some rodents) are seen in the emergency setting and require treatment similar to the treatment of dog and cat bites. One should obtain a careful history about the event that caused the bite and the location and type of the animal because these bites carry a higher risk for rabies. Usually, if the animal is not observable or if the bite was unprovoked, rabies prophylaxis is indicated. If the animal exhibited signs of rabies at the time of exposure, rabies treatment should begin as soon as possible. One should consult with the local health department or an infectious disease specialist if there is a question about the need for rabies treatment.

Up to four cases of human rabies are reported each year in the United States. The incubation period for rabies is between 10 days and 8 weeks. For postexposure prophylaxis following animal bite, both the antirabies globulin and the vaccine are recommended.

SNAKE BITES

General Information

Bites sustained from nonvenomous snakes and venomous crotalid snakes (rattlesnakes, copperheads, cottonmouths, water moccasins, pit vipers) are common emergency room problems in certain areas of the United States.

Diagnostic Criteria

History

If the patient is conscious, determine the time of envenomation and the specific sites of envenomation. Assess the general pain level and loss of sensation or function. If it is determined that the patient has been bitten by a crotalid species (pit viper), then the specific type of snake is not important. Determine the date of last tetanus immunization and ask specifically about allergies to horse serum. A small number of snakebites in the United States occur from elapid snakes (coral snakes and exotic snakes not indigenous to North America). Elapid snakebite envenomation often requires different treatment than does crotalid envenomation because the snake venom has a different mechanism of action.

Physical Examination

General physical examination should focus on changes that would be consistent with systemic effects of crotalid venom. Blood pressure, mental status, and other general findings should be recorded. Noncardiogenic pulmonary edema, renal failure, and systemic coagulopathy have been reported.

One should examine the specific site of envenomation and record the separation of fang marks, level of contamination, and amount of swelling. Two discrete puncture wounds are consistent with crotalid envenomation. The bites are tender and often surrounded by an area of ecchymosis. The depth of envenomation is usually twice the interfang distance. These data can help predict the risk of intracompartmental envenomation. The limb should be examined to assess specifically for unusual amounts of swelling, neurologic deficiency, or compartment syndrome.

Other Assessment

Laboratory studies should be done to assess systemic evidence of envenomation further. A complete blood count, platelet count, general chemistries, a coagulation profile, and a urinalysis should be done if a question exists of systemic effect from envenomation.

A chest x-ray, electrocardiogram, arterial blood gas, and tests for serum fibrinogen and fibrin split products should be ordered if evidence exists of severe envenomation.

Compartment pressure measurements should be done if limb swelling is severe. The signs of envenomation and compartment syndrome are similar. Objective evaluation of compartment pressures can help guide further treatment. In general, compartment syndrome following crotalid envenomation is uncommon.

Differential Diagnosis

The most important part of the differential diagnosis is to make sure that the patient identified a snake as being responsible for the bite and that the snake was a crotalid. Nonvenomous snakebites do not have characteristic fang marks. Elapid snakes (coral snakes) bite using a different mechanism and also require different antivenin. Their colorful rings often identify coral snakes. (The mnemonic is, "Red on yellow kill a fellow, red on black venom lack.") Elapid envenomations are much less common than crotalid envenomations. Bites from nonvenomous snakes also do not require antivenin.

Grading Envenomation

0   Snakebite without envenomation ("dry bite")
1   Mild envenomation: local changes, no limb edema
2   Moderate envenomation: limb edema beyond the site of the bite, progressive swelling, one or more systemic abnormalities; laboratory parameters may be abnormal
3   Severe envenomation: marked local response, severe systemic alterations, and significant alteration in laboratory findings

Treatment

Initial treatment of the local bite wound requires local irrigation and débridement of the wound and the application of a dressing that immobilizes the hand in a functional position. If necessary, a tetanus toxoid should be administered. The patient is begun on a first-generation cephalosporin. If limb edema is severe, then measurement of compartment pressures should be done. Nonvenomous snakebites usually only require this method of local care.

The intravenous administration of crotalidae antivenin should be considered if evidence exists of severe progressive limb symptoms or systemic envenomation. Because of the possibility of an anaphylactic reaction to antivenin, patients receiving antivenin should be carefully monitored. Before the administration of antivenin, one should place intravenous lines sufficient for the purposes of resuscitation. For mild envenomation, zero to four vials of antivenin should be used; for moderate envenomation, four to seven vials; and for severe envenomation, 15 or more vials are needed.

KEY POINTS

- Approximately 25% of all snakebites are dry (or are not associated with envenomation).
- Typically, rattlesnakebites are more severe than bites from cottonmouths or copperheads.
- Bites on the digit are difficult to assess and are often associated with full-thickness skin loss.
- No benefit to venom extraction methods (Sawyer suction device) exists 30 minutes after envenomation.
- One should consider consultation with a toxicologist. A call to the local or regional poison control center is warranted to obtain specific protocols for managing a snakebite.

SPIDER BITES: BROWN RECLUSE

General Information

The brown recluse spider (Loxosceles reclusa) is found throughout the southern United States. These spiders prefer dark outdoor areas (wood piles) and can be as large as 6 cm in size. The brown recluse spider is characterized by a brown "fiddle" on its back. The Loxosceles spiders secrete proteolytic venom that can cause significant local tissue destruction and have a severe systemic effect.

Following envenomation, systemic toxicity (arachnidism) may develop before the onset of local symptoms. In general, the severity of the bite is determined by the location of the bite, amount of envenomation, and status of the host.

Diagnostic Criteria

History

Patients usually describe a bite that becomes tender and swollen. Often the spider has not been directly identified and the time of the bite is uncertain.

Physical Examination

In severe envenomations, patients may present with fever, malaise, myalgia, arthralgia, coagulopathy, nausea, and vomiting. The local lesion is characterized by a tender purpuric bleb. Local tissue necrosis may occur within hours.

Other Assessment

Patients with evidence of systemic arachnidism should have a thorough general medical evaluation. Laboratory assessment should include a CBC, platelet count, PT, PTT, fibrinogen, and fibrin split products.

Differential Diagnosis

The necrotic lesion that is characterizes the brown recluse spider bite can be produced by a number of spiders, venomous ants, and fish.

Treatment

Initial local treatment focuses on cleansing the lesion and local wound care. Tetanus status should be updated when appropriate. A first-generation cephalosporin is usually administered.

Oral use of Dapsone and Colchicine may prevent lesion ulceration if administered early. Dapsone is contraindicated in patients with a G6PD deficiency.

For patients with systemic arachnidism, consult a toxicologist or infectious disease specialist. Systemic arachnidism usually requires significant systemic support, using intravenous fluids, corticosteroids, and treatment of coagulopathy.

KEY POINTS

- Significant ulcerations may take months to heal.
- Local wound cleansing and dressing changes are the best treatment for the local lesions.

SPIDER BITES: BLACK WIDOW

General Information

Black widow spiders (Lactrodectus mactans) are indigenous to many areas of North America. Almost all significant envenomations occur from female spider bites. The black widow spider is shiny black with a red hourglass on the ventral surface of the spider. Significant regional variation occurs in the appearance of these spiders (red widow: Lactrodectus bishopi; brown widow: Lactrodectus geometricus).

Diagnostic Criteria

History

Most patients describe the bite as a painful needlelike sensation.

Physical Examination

The wound characteristic of a black widow envenomation is two minute puncture wounds surrounded by a halo. The inner ring of the halo is white and the outer ring is red. Multiple bites are common.

Treatment

Initial treatment is open-wound management. Tetanus immunization should be updated when appropriate. Patients usually require significant treatment for pain. Lactrodectus mactans horse sera antivenin is available for the treatment of severe envenomations. As with all horse sera products, skin testing is recommended before administration. Appropriate life-support systems should be available.

KEY POINTS

- Deaths are rare with appropriate supportive care.
- Black widow spiders secrete a cholinergic venom that induces muscle cramping, diaphoresis, salivation, headache, nausea, and vomiting.
- Venom effects peak at 18 hours following envenomation.
- Symptoms may last for 3 weeks.
- The "halo lesion" is very suggestive of a black widow spider bite.

SCORPION BITES

General Information

Although several different types of scorpions are capable of stinging, envenomation injuries from the bark scorpion (Centruroides sculpturatus) are the most severe. The bark scorpion is a small (3 mm to 1 cm) light-brown animal that stings from its sixth and last tail segment (the telson). Scorpions prefer dark areas and warm weather. They inhabit palm trees, sycamore trees, mesquite, and cottonwood.

Diagnostic Criteria

History

Often patients will not have seen the scorpion but have a history of environmental exposure that could be consistent with animal envenomation. The bites produce significant and immediate local pain. Patients may describe symptoms of increased parasympathetic tone (thick tongue, nausea).

Physical Examination

Patients with more severe envenomations present with tachycardia, excessive secretions, blurred vision, roving eye movements, and muscular fasciculations. Although no lesion may be visible, tapping at the site of envenomation often produces severe pain. Significant paresthesias are often associated with the bite.

Grading Envenomation

I   Local pain at the site
II   Pain and/or paresthesias remote from the site of envenomation
III One cranial or somatic neuromuscular symptom
IV   Two or more cranial and somatic neuromuscular symptoms

Treatment

All patients with scorpion bites should be observed in the emergency room for progression of symptoms. Patients who have moderate to severe envenomations may require the intravenous administration of goat serum antivenin (developed for Centruroides sculpturatus) and should be seen by a toxicologist or critical care specialist. The antivenin is effective in helping to control systemic manifestations of envenomation but does not have a significant effect on local pain or paresthesias.

Patients need local care and oral analgesics for the envenomation site. When necessary, tetanus immunization status should be updated.

KEY POINTS

- Bark scorpions (Centruroides sculpturatus), found in California, Nevada, Arizona, Texas, and New Mexico, can produce severe envenomation injuries and life-threatening illness.

- The venom of the bark scorpion is a complex protein substance that produces primarily neurologic effects. Scorpion venom binds sodium channels in neurons causing prolonged activation of parasympathetic, sympathetic, and somatic neurons.
- Death from scorpion bites is very rare in the United States. Most severe envenomations are seen in children less than 10 years of age.
- Envenomation from scorpions indigenous to other countries can be associated with severe systemic symptoms (adrenergic storm) and death.

29

Dupuytren's Disease

GENERAL INFORMATION

Dupuytren's disease is a condition of the hand that replaces normal digital and palmar fascia (bands and sheaths) with abnormal fibrous tissue (nodules and cords) consisting of immature fibroblasts, myofibroblasts, and Type III collagen. Dupuytren's disease is particularly common in people of Northern European descent and is associated with alcoholism, smoking, diabetes mellitus, and the use of anticonvulsant medications. The condition is rare in children; its incidence increases with age (40 to 60 years of age). It is also seen more commonly in men and frequently involves both hands. Some patients may have a more aggressive form of the disease (diathesis), and are noted to have a strong family history, early onset of the disease, bilateral hand involvement, and ectopic deposits (foot and penile involvement).

DIAGNOSTIC CRITERIA

Often, patients present for evaluation of "lumps" (nodules) in the palm, which may or may not be painful. More commonly, they have progressive, painless flexion contractures of the metacarpophalangeal and proximal interphalangeal joints, and occasionally, the distal interphalangeal joint. Contractures of the ring and small finger are the most common, although the thumb, thumb web space, and other digits also can be affected.

Physical Examination

Patients have palmar nodules, which may or may not be tender. Longitudinally oriented diseased cords are palpable on the palmar aspect of fingers (Fig. 1). Web space cords may be transversely oriented. Thickenings over the dorsal aspect of the metacarpophalangeal joints (knuckle pads or Garrod's nodes) may be present (Fig. 1). Similar changes may be found on the sole of the foot (Lederhosen's disease) and the penis (Peyronie's disease).

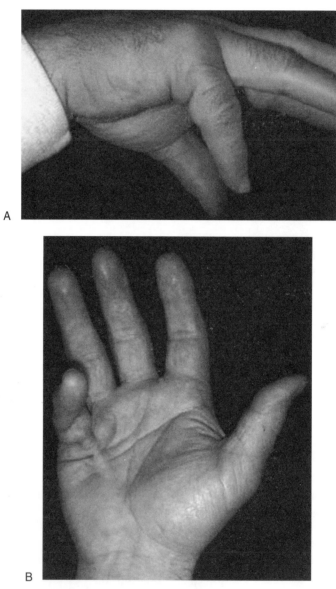

FIG. 1. A: Typical appearance of a patient's hand with Dupuytren's contracture. **B:** Dupuytren's fibrosis causing a fixed flexion deformity of the metacarpophalangeal joint and the proximal interphalangeal joint.

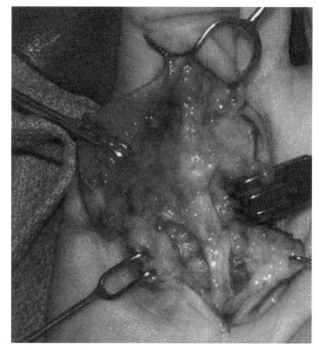

C

FIG. 1 *(continued).* **C:** Operative appearance of Dupuytren's fascia.

TREATMENT

The early management of mild Dupuytren's contracture is observation, reassurance, and periodic reexaminations. Nonoperative treatment to date has not proven effective in treating progressive Dupuytren's disease. Steroid and particularly enzyme injections may prove useful in the future.

The indications for the surgical management of Dupuytren's contracture include a metacarpophalangeal joint flexion contracture greater than 30 degrees. Surgery for any contractures involving PIPS is recommended by some authors because of the difficulty of maintaining correction of a proximal interphalangeal joint flexion contracture.

The surgical options for treating digital flexion contractures include fasciotomy (simply cutting the diseased cord), segmental fasciotomy (partial removal of the diseased cord), selective fasciotomy (removal of all diseased cords and fascia), and radical fasciectomy (removal of all palmar fascia) (Fig. 1). The surgical management of the skin includes direct skin closure, full-thickness skin grafting, or an open wound technique.

It is essential to preserve finger flexion while attempting to improve the finger extension gained with surgery. Hand therapists are frequently employed during the postoperative recovery period. Finger flexion should be initiated immediately when skin grafts are not used; and as soon as the skin grafts have healed, when grafts have been used to cover skin defects. Twice-daily dressing changes with saline-dampened gauze are used to promote healing for those incisions left open to heal with granulation tissue. Healed incisions can be massaged with cocoa butter and vitamin E oil. Silicone patches may help soften scarred areas. Early use of "static" splints may help maintain finger extension, but should be used judiciously to ensure that finger flexion is not compromised.

Correction is usually maintained at the metacarpophalangeal joint level. Persistent or recurrent contractures of the proximal interphalangeal joint are common. Recurrence rates vary from 26% to 80%. Treatment of recurrent disease can involve a dermofasciectomy (removal of diseased fascia and overlying skin) followed by full-thickness skin grafting.

SELECTED REFERENCES

Badalamente MA, Hurst LC. Enzyme injection as nonsurgical treatment of Dupuytren's disease. J Hand Surg 2000;25A:629–636.

Hueston JT. Dupuytren's contracture. E&S Livingston Ltd, Edinburgh, 1963.

Hurst L, Starkweather KD, Badalamente MA. Dupuytren's disease. In: Peimer C, ed. Surgery of the hand and upper extremity. McGraw-Hill, New York, 1996, pp. 1601–1615.

McFarlane RM. Patterns of the diseased fascia in the fingers in Dupuytren's contracture. Plast Reconstr Surg 1974;54:31–44.

McGrouther DA. Dupuytren's contracture. In: Green DP, Hotchkiss RN, Pederson WC, eds. Green's operative hand surgery, 4th ed. Churchill Livingstone, 1999, pp. 563–603.

30

Congenital Anomalies

Congenital anomalies of the upper extremity occur in approximately one out of 626 live births. The most widely accepted clinical classification of congenital limb anomalies was adopted by the American Society for Surgery of the Hand, International Federation of Societies for Surgery of the Hand, and International Society for Prosthetics and Orthotics. This work was designed to organize anomalies according to embryonic failure during development. This classification relies on the clinical diagnosis, and each limb malformation is categorized into one of seven categories according to its predominant anomaly (Table 1). Different clinical presentations of similar categories are explained by varying degrees of damage during embryogenesis.

Group I is divided into transverse or longitudinal failure of formation. Transverse deficiencies are also called congenital amputations and are termed according to the anatomic level of limb termination. The most common site of amputation occurs at the proximal third of the forearm (Fig. 1). Rudimentary digits can be located on the end of the amputation stump. A fetal vascular insult to the developing limb is the most prevalent explanation for these deficiencies. Early chorionic villous sampling and failed attempts at pregnancy termination by dilatation and curettage have been associated with transverse limb deficiencies.

Longitudinal deficiencies are named according to bones that are partially or completely absent. These deficiencies can be divided into radial (preaxial), ulnar (postaxial), or central forms. The central type includes deficiencies of the index, long, and ring rays (digits and underlying carpus). The typical cleft hand has a V-shaped deficiency involving at least the long ray (Fig. 2). This type is often bilateral, familial, and includes the feet. In contrast, an atypical cleft deformity is also known as symbrachydactyly and has a U-shaped deficiency. The extent and number of affected digits are variable and can range from mild deficiencies of the central rays to a monodactylous or adactylous hand. This type is usually unilateral, nonfamilial, and without involvement of the feet.

Radial deficiencies are approximately ten times more common than their ulnar complement. Exposure to teratogens such as thalidomide and radiation can cause radial deficiencies, although the majority of cases are sporadic without

TABLE 1. *Embryologic classification of congenital anomalies*

Classification	Subheading	Subgroup	Category
Failure of formation			
	Transverse arrest		
		Shoulder	
		Arm	
		Elbow	
		Forearm	
		Wrist	
		Carpal	
		Metacarpal	
		Phalanx	
	Longitudinal arrest		
		Radial deficiency	
		Ulnar deficiency	
		Central deficiency	
		Intersegmental	Phocomelia
Failure of differentiation			
	Soft tissue		
		Dissemenated	Arthrogryposis
		Shoulder	
		Elbow and forearm	
		Wrist and hand	Cutaneous syndactyly
			Camptodactyly
			Thumb-in-palm
			Deviated deformed digits
	Skeletal		
		Shoulder	
		Elbow	Synostosis
		Forearm	Proximal
			Distal
		Wrist and hand	Osseous syndactyly
			Carpal bone synsostosis
			Symphalangia
			Clinodactyly
	Tumorous conditions		
		Hemangiotic	
		Lymphatic	
		Neurogenic	
		Connective tissue	
		Skeletal	
Duplication			
	Whole limb		
	Humeral		
	Radial		
	Ulnar		
		Mirror hand	
	Digit		
		Polydactyly	Radial (preaxial)
			Central
			Ulnar (postaxial)
Overgrowth			
	Whole limb		
	Partial limb		
	Digit		
		Macrodactyly	

TABLE 1 *(continued).*

Classification	Subheading	Subgroup	Category
Undergrowth			
	Whole limb		
	Whole hand		
	Metacarpal		
	Digit		
		Brachysyndactyly	
		Brachydactyly	
Constriction band syndrome			
Generalized skeletal abnormalities			

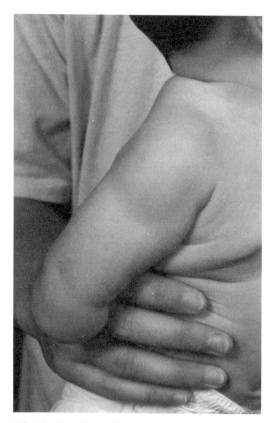

FIG. 1. Child with a short below-the-elbow congenital amputation.

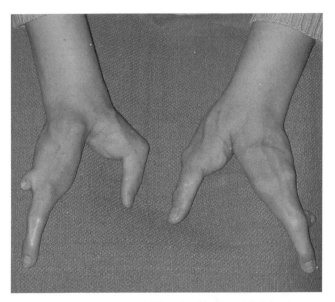

FIG. 2. Bilateral typical cleft hands with central deficiencies.

any definable cause. Of all radial deficiencies, 50% are bilateral. The types vary depending on the amount of radius missing. The most common form has a complete absence of the radius and is often associated with thumb hypoplasia. The remaining ulna is always decreased in length (approximately 60% of normal). This discrepancy persists throughout the growth period. The ulna is thickened and frequently bowed toward the absent radius. The wrist is positioned in radial deviation and eventually becomes perpendicular to the forearm (Fig. 3). Radial deficiency is associated with numerous syndromes; the most common are Holt-Oram (cardiac septal defects), TAR (thrombocytopenia, absent radius), Fanconi's anemia (aplastic anemia), and VACTERL (vertebral, anal, cardiac, tracheoesophageal, renal, and limb abnormalities). These syndromes require appropriate evaluation in any child with a radial deficiency.

Early intervention is recommended for children with radial deficiencies and consists of passive stretching of the taught radial structures performed at each diaper change and bedtime. A forearm-based splint is fabricated to prevent progressive radial deviation. Surgical centralization of the wrist on the ulna remains the standard treatment to correct the radial deviation. This surgery is performed at about 1 year of age. The carpus is reduced onto the distal ulna and tendon transfers are performed to balance the carpus. Surgery should be avoided in children with a limited life expectancy (e.g., aplastic anemia), mild deformity with adequate support for the hand, an elbow extension contracture that prevents the hand from reaching the mouth, and in adults who have adjusted to their deformity. Thumb hypoplasia is usually addressed at a second stage after wrist centralization.

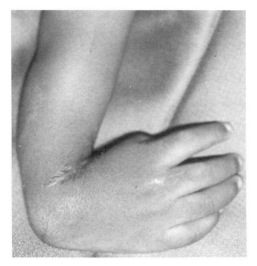

FIG. 3. Wrist positioned perpendicular to the forearm in a child with radial deficiency.

Thumb hypoplasia is usually addressed at a second stage after wrist centralization. Group II category includes failure of differentiation or separation of parts. This grouping implies development of all the essential components, but failure of arrangement into a proper finalized form. This failure of differentiation can affect skeletal, dermal, fascial, muscular, ligaments, and/or neurovascular components of the limb. Syndactyly is the most common presentation of a group II anomaly and occurs with an incidence of approximately two to three per 10,000 live births (Fig. 4). Heritable, spontaneous, and syndromic forms have

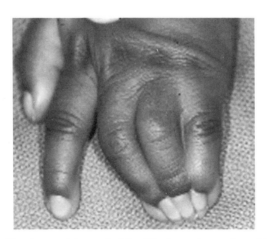

FIG. 4. Simple complete syndactyly of the long, ring, and small fingers.

TABLE 2. *Properties of syndactyly*

Type	Characteristics
Simple	Soft tissue alone
Complex	Soft tissue and bone
Incomplete	Partial connection between digits
Complete	Complete connection between digits
Complicated	Extensive soft-tissue abnormalities or a hodgepodge of abnormal bones

Syndactyly can be defined using multiple types (e.g., simple and incomplete).

been identified with various similarities and dissimilarities. Heritable syndactylism is associated with a genetic defect involving particular candidate regions on the second chromosome. The mode of transmission is considered to be autosomal dominant with variable expressivity and incomplete penetrance. This terminology implies familial propagation, although the syndactyly may skip a generation (incomplete penetrance) and not be present in full form (variable phenotype). The extent of digital union is variable and defined according to certain characteristics (Table 2). The treatment of syndactyly involves separation of the connected digits as long as the digits will function as independent entities. Syndactyly separation follows established principles with regard to timing, technique, and postoperative management. Early release of border digits is required to promote function and prevent contracture. Proper flap design provides com-

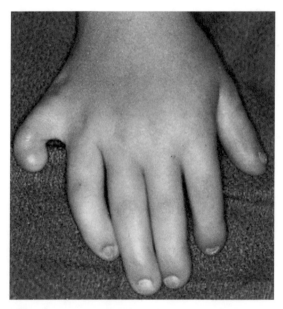

FIG. 5. Postaxial polydactyly with a well-formed ulnar digit.

missure reconstruction and avoids the use of skin graft within the web space. Identification of neurovascular anomalies and preservation of critical vascular inflow maintains digital perfusion. Postoperative dressings provide compression to skin grafted areas and protection to the underlying digits. Adherence to recognized principles yields acceptable results, although complications can emerge requiring additional treatment.

Group III anomalies represent duplication of parts and are most commonly observed as polydactyly. Postaxial (ulnar-sided) polydactyly is commonly inherited (autosomal dominant) and is more common in African-American than white children (Fig. 5). The digit can be extremely hypoplastic and connected via a small pedicle. This type of polydactyly can be treated with suture ligation of the pedicle in the nursery. The digit will eventually become gangrenous and fall off. Well-formed polydactyly requires formal reconstruction with reorganization of any important collateral ligaments or muscles (e.g., abductor digiti minimi) that attach to the ablated digit. Preaxial duplication (radial-sided) is more common in white children, but is usually unilateral and sporadic. This duplication requires removal of the smaller part and reconstruction of the retained component.

Group IV abnormalities are listed as overgrowth and can be manifested as diffuse hypertrophy of the entire limb or isolated enlargement of various parts (Fig. 6). This category is uncommon in occurrence, but dramatic in presentation. Underlying causes for limb overgrowth (e.g., vascular abnormalities or malformations) must be considered during patient evaluation. In addition, overgrowth

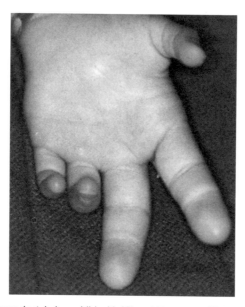

FIG. 6. Macrodactyly in a child with Klippel-Trenaunay-Weber syndrome.

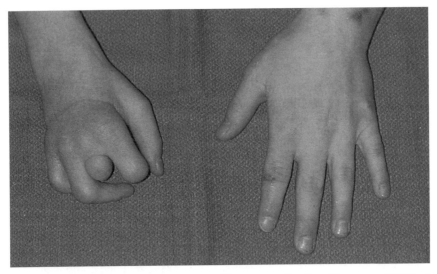

FIG. 7. Amniotic disruption sequence of the right upper extremity with a constriction band around the hand and loss of the long digit.

can be a constituent of a variety of syndromes (e.g., neurofibromatosis or Klippel-Trenaunay-Weber syndrome). Treatment depends on the extent of limb involvement, size of affected part(s), and the presence or absence of progressive enlargement.

Group V deformities correspond to undergrowth or hypoplasia of the limb or its parts. The manifestations of hypoplasia are subdivided according to anatomic location. Hypoplasia is prevalent in many disorders. For example, ipsilateral hand hypoplasia associated with chest wall deficiencies is typical in children with Poland's syndrome.

Group VI anomalies occur with constriction band syndrome (amniotic disruption sequence). These deficiencies are not hereditary and the cause remains controversial. Amniotic bands cause digital damage, which initiates an embryonic repair process, which in turn causes a variable amount of circumferential stricture. Severe damage can lead to complete vascular ischemia and complete truncation of the affected part(s) (Fig. 7).

SELECTED REFERENCES

Bayne LG, Klug MS. Long-term review of the surgical treatment of radial deficiencies. J Hand Surg 1987;12:169–179.

Damore E, Kozin SH, Thoder JJ, Porter S. The recurrence of deformity after surgical centralization for radial clubhand. J Hand Surg 2000;25A:745–751.

Flatt AE. Classification and incidence. In: The care of congenital hand anomalies, 2nd ed. Quality Medical Publishing, St. Louis, MO, 1994, pp. 47–63.

Heikel HVA. Aplasia and hypoplasia of the radius. Studies on 64 cases and on epiphyseal transplantation in rabbits with the imitated defect. Acta Orthop Scand 1959;39:1–155.

Kozin SH. Syndactyly. J Am Soc Surg Hand 2001;1:1–13.

Manske PR, McCarroll HR Jr, James MA. Type III-A hypoplastic thumb. J Hand Surg 1995;20A: 246–253.

McCarroll HR. Congenital anomalies: a 25-year overview. J Hand Surg 2000;25A:1007–1037.

Swanson AB. A classification for congenital limb malformations. J Hand Surg 1976;1:8–22.

Watson BT, Hennrikus WL. Postaxial type-B polydactyly. Prevalence and treatment. J Bone Joint Surg Am 1997;79:65–68.

31

Amputations

GENERAL INFORMATION

Upper extremity amputations are common injuries. Rates of limb salvage have increased during the last 20 years with improvements in microvascular techniques. Any patient desiring replantation should be referred to an appropriate facility. One should never promise the patient that replantation is possible. Patients are treated individually based on the nature and level of injury, associated medical conditions, time that has elapsed since the injury, and the patient's personal desires.

By definition, replantation is a reattachment of a body part that has been totally severed from the body (complete amputation). A revascularization is reconstruction of blood vessels that have been damaged in order to prevent an ischemic body part from becoming nonviable or necrotic (incomplete amputation).

DIAGNOSTIC CRITERIA

On initial assessment and treatment, the patient must be given realistic expectations about whether the injured part can be salvaged. In general, the indications for replantation include amputation of a thumb, multiple digits, or a limb through the forearm, wrist, or palm. Amputations through the elbow and proximal arm should only be replanted if the part is a sharp amputation or has minimal crush injury. Single digits distal to the insertion of the flexor digitorum profundus (FDP) tendon in the middle phalanx may be replanted in appropriate patients. A child with almost any body part amputated is a candidate, although the success rate of replantation in children is lower.

Contraindications include severely crushed or mangled parts, amputations at multiple levels, prolonged ischemic times, and amputations in patients with other serious injuries or medical illnesses. A variety of conditions may complicate limb reconstruction, including diabetes, peripheral vascular disease, smoking, or previous trauma to the affected limb. Individual fingers in adults amputated proximal to the insertion of the FDP tendon should not be replanted because of the poor functional results that are obtained.

When the patient is being transferred from another institution, appropriate care of the patient and part must begin with the transferring institution. The part should be wrapped in gauze moistened with Ringer's lactate or normal saline. This is placed into a plastic bag and sealed. The bag is then immersed into ice water (Fig. 1). The patient needs to be initially assessed and stabilized for transfer. A pressure dressing is applied to the stump. No attempt should be made to ligate bleeding vessels.

On arrival, a complete trauma assessment is required, particularly in amputations proximal to the wrist. Evaluation starts with the ABCs of resuscitation and includes assessment for associated injuries such as ipsilateral brachial plexus and cervical spine injuries.

The patient can be considered a candidate for replantation or revascularization after initial stabilization. The ischemia time should not exceed 6 hours when a significant amount of muscle is included in the amputated part. Digits that have been cooled have been successfully replanted up to 24 hours after amputation. In cases of incomplete amputation, perfusion via intact skin/muscle will extend the period of time that successful revascularization is possible. In all injuries, examination includes signs of tissue damage at sites remote from the site of amputation (e.g., segmental vessel injury, crush injury, burns, and evidence of tendon or nerve avulsion). The "ribbon sign," a digital artery with multiple folds, is a sign of an avulsion injury. The "red stripe sign" is intramural hemorrhage in the walls of the digital vessel. Both of these indicate a lower chance of saving the injured part.

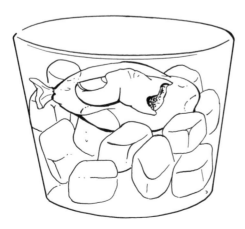

FIG. 1. Care of amputated part.

In partial amputations, assessment of circulation includes color, turgor, capillary refill, and pulses. Skin bridges may supply adequate venous drainage. Motor and sensory function of distal parts should be assessed.

With improved microsurgical techniques, it is possible to restore circulation to most devascularized extremities. It is the surgeon's responsibility to provide a realistic "preview" of what the patient will have to endure in surgery and during the postoperative period and what he or she can expect to gain.

Other Assessments

Radiographs of the limb and the amputated part should be obtained to plan fixation of the fractures.

TREATMENT

In the operating room, vascular spasm is minimized with an axillary block, preferably with a catheter, and by keeping the patient warm. In major limb replantations, a central line should be placed for fluid resuscitation and transfusions.

The general surgical order is adequate exposure and identification of nerves and vessels, appropriate débridement, shortening and fixation of the bone, repair of extensor tendons, repair of flexor tendons, repair of arteries, repair of nerves, repair of veins, and loose closure of the skin (Table 1). Ideally, two veins should be repaired for each artery.

AFTERCARE

Replanted or revascularized limbs should be splinted and wrapped in nonconstrictive dressings. Monitoring of the limb or digit is accomplished with frequent examination for color, turgor, and capillary refill. Temperature or pulse oximetry probes can be used for continuous monitoring. Patients are anticoagulated with aspirin, heparin, or Dextran.

TABLE 1. *Treatment priorities*

Indications for replantation	Relative contraindications to replantation	Contraindications
Amputations proximal to the wrist	Mechanism of severe crushing or avulsion	Severe associated injuries
Amputation of multiple digits	Single digit amputations in adults, particularly in zone 2	Multilevel major limb amputations
Thumb amputations	Heavy wound contamination	Other serious diseases or injuries
Pediatric amputations	Psychiatric disease with willful self-amputation	

The failing replant is signaled by a change in color and temperature. Pallor, with loss of capillary refill, is a sign of arterial insufficiency. A replanted part becomes blue and swollen when venous drainage is insufficient. Constrictive dressings should be loosened. In some cases of venous congestion, treatment consists of removing the nail and placing a medicinal leech on the exposed nail bed. The leech mechanically decompresses the congested part and secretes a protein anticoagulant (hirudin).

There is a risk of postoperative lactic acidosis and myoglobinuria in major limb replantation and revascularization where there has been an extended period of ischemia. The patient should be well hydrated, and urine output should be carefully monitored. Serial blood gases are followed; sodium bicarbonate may be necessary to alkalinize the serum and urine.

Extensive rehabilitation is necessary following replantation. Often patients require several surgical procedures, a week of hospitalization, and several months of occupational therapy. Stiffness, loss of sensation, lack of strength, and cold intolerance often complicate replantations. Maximum medical improvement may take over a year.

SELECTED REFERENCES

Graham B, Adkins P, Tsai T-M, et al. Major replantation versus revision amputation and prosthetic fitting in the upper extremity: a late functional outcomes study. J Hand Surg 1998;23A:783–791.

Urbaniak JR, Roth JH, Nunley JA, et al. The results of replantation after amputation of a single finger. J Bone Joint Surg 1985;67A:611–9.

Weinzweig N, Sharzer LA, Starker I. Replantation and revascularization at the transmetacarpal level: long-term functional results. J Hand Surg 1996;21A:877–883.

32

Nail Bed and Fingertip Injuries

GENERAL INFORMATION

Fingertip injuries are the most common trauma in the hand, accounting for up to 50% of emergency room visits for hand care. Traditional treatment was shortening and closure by any possible method. Goals for repair of the injured fingertip include identification and cleaning of injured structures, maintenance of bone length, and meticulous repair of the soft-tissue envelope.

DIAGNOSTIC CRITERIA

Most fingertip injuries occur as low-energy crush injuries such as those produced by closing a door on the digit. Although tissue is disrupted, it is not usually missing (Fig. 1). More powerful crushing injuries from mechanical presses devitalize tissue and may need extensive débridement. Slicing injuries amputate tissue cleanly and may be suitable for replantation. Ripping injuries from power saws combine crushing and slicing and often produce large-tissue defects requiring graft or flap coverage. A brief health assessment should include medical problems, medications, and allergies.

Physical Examination

Identification of the injured structures is critical for repair. Patients present with painful, bleeding digits. After a brief sensory examination, a digital block will relieve pain (anesthesia section). A digital tourniquet controls bleeding and can be fashioned from a 1/2-in. Penrose drain. Physical examination includes an assessment of vascularity in partial amputations. Skin, nail bed, bone, and tendon may be involved, which are often not initially visible on primary inspection. Irrigation with saline and peroxide removes clot and allows visual inspection. X-rays should focus on the injured finger and not the entire hand. Subtle bony injuries are missed when the beam is not centered on the digit. X-rays may also demonstrate soft-tissue defects exposing bone and foreign bodies that require removal.

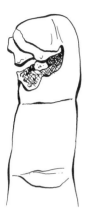

FIG. 1. Incomplete fingertip amputation.

TREATMENT

Clear communication with consulting surgeons regarding the nature of the injury, including which tissues are injured, helps guide treatment. Accurate descriptions of bone, nail bed, and pulp injuries facilitate appropriate treatment. Most fingertip injuries can be treated in a well equipped emergency department. Pulp hematomas occur when crushing energy is not strong enough to produce open injuries. Nevertheless, pressure from blood within the pulp produces a painful swollen digit. The cavities between the fibrous septate of the pulp rapidly fill with blood. A nondisplaced tuft fracture is often present. Treatment of these injuries may be purely supportive with analgesics and splints. Alternatively, sterile aspiration of the hematoma and instillation of 0.5 mL bupivacaine relieves pain significantly for 6 to 12 hours. Subungual hematomas of less than 30% of the nail bed also may be treated symptomatically. Drainage of the hematoma using a heated paperclip, 18-gauge needle, or ophthalmic cautery relieves pressure and pain.

Nail bed lacerations are common in incomplete amputations (Fig. 2). These injuries require a bloodless field for identification and repair of injured tissue.

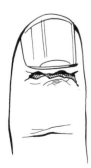

FIG. 2. Laceration at origin of nail matrix.

The injured digit should be gently scrubbed with a Betadine or chlorhexidine scrub. Dirt or metal fragments can be removed with a sterile toothbrush or dental pick. An arm board allows the finger to be draped away from the body. The injured nail plate is removed from the nail fold. The wound is irrigated with 500 cc of saline and residual clot and foreign material are removed. Grossly unstable metaphyseal fractures of the distal phalanx are stabilized with a small wire. Battery powered drivers are ideal for pin placement. A 19- or 20-gauge needle driven in with a 10-cc syringe also provides stability. The nail bed injury is defined and repaired with 6-0 or 7-0 absorbable suture. Proximal injuries require dorsal oblique incisions of the nail fold for visualization and repair. Power tool injuries often result in loss of nail bed tissue. Partial-thickness nail bed may be harvested from the same or adjoining digit to fill the defect and prevent loss of nail adherence. Injured pulp tissue is repaired with 4-0 or 5-0 nonabsorbable suture.

Following repair of the nail bed, the nail fold must be stented open to allow nail regeneration. Minimally injured nails placed within the nail fold will often "take" and not extrude later with nail growth. Alternative materials used as nail fold stents include nonadherent gauze, foil from a suture package, or silicon sheets.

COMPLETE AMPUTATIONS

Complete amputations of the fingertip distal to the flexor tendon insertion present the additional challenge of devascularized tissue (Fig. 3). Thin skin and nail bed avulsions (1 to 2 mm) survive well when repaired primarily. Thicker skin and subcutaneous tissue loss without exposed bone heal well by secondary intention. This allows wound contraction to decrease insensate areas often found following skin grafting.

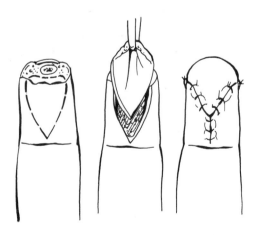

FIG. 3. Complete fingertip amputation with V-Y flap repair.

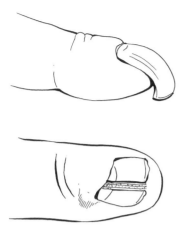

FIG. 4. Hook/split nail.

Exposed bone following amputation presents a reconstructive challenge. The broad tuft of the distal phalanx is essential to a normal flat nail. Shortening of the distal phalanx may lead to a hooked nail especially if residual nail bed is sutured palmar to the plane of the nail (Fig. 4). Should primary shortening of the nail occur, the nail bed should be shortened to the level of the residual bone and palmar tissue brought dorsally for final coverage.

Flap coverage of the fingertip is primary alternative to bone shortening. Local V-Y advancement flaps from palmar or lateral tissue can be advanced up to 1 cm. Larger defects require distant flaps such as a cross finger or thenar. Newer vascular pedicled and free flaps for the fingertip provide excellent coverage, yet are technically challenging.

POSTOPERATIVE CARE

A course of antibiotics over 3 days is recommended postoperatively for injuries involving the distal phalanx. A bulky sterile bandage covers the fingertip for 7 to 10 days unless vascular monitoring is needed. If possible, early mobilization of the metaphalangeal and proximal interphalangeal joints prevents significant digital stiffness. Washing with soap and water begins at 2 weeks and may be supplemented by skin softeners to decrease scar formation and tip sensitivity. Moldable plastic splints provide protection and early return to functional use of the digit. Hand therapy for decreased mobility and tip sensitivity may speed recovery.

Results following fingertip injury vary with the severity of the initial injury. More distal, low-energy injuries may return 100% function. More proximal injuries and amputations demonstrate some residual stiffness and cold sensitivity, which decreases with time. Revision surgery is indicated for ingrown or prominent nail remnants. Wide excision and full thickness skin grafting decrease recurrence. Painful neuromas exacerbated by pinch can be transposed dorsally to improve function.

SELECTED REFERENCES

Ashbell TS, et al. The deformed fingernail, a frequent result of failure to repair nail bed injuries. J Trauma 1967;7:177–190.

Foucher G, Khouri RK. Digital reconstruction with island flaps. Clin Plas Surg 1997;24:1–32.

Zook EG, et al. Anatomy and physiology of the perionychium: a review of the literature and anatomic study. J Hand Surg 1980;5:528–536.

33

Foreign Bodies

GENERAL INFORMATION

Typical foreign bodies (FB) include implants used in surgery as well as more obvious foreign agents such as thorns, pencil leads, and bullets. The FB itself may be less of an issue than the material on or within it. An example would be a hollow-bore needle carrying a viral contaminant. Thus, the examiner considering the diagnosis and management of an FB should begin by identifying these key characteristics:

- Does the agent contain or release noxious chemicals (e.g., lead, mercury, etc)?
- Does the agent carry a potential infectious agent(s)?
- Is the agent in a damaging or potentially damaging location?

DIAGNOSTIC CRITERIA

History

The patient usually recalls a direct injury. For example, a worker using a high-pressure paint gun will likely state, "I was using the 'paint gun' when it was bumped and touched my opposite hand. I felt a stabbing pain into my arm immediately."

In any work- or accident-related injury, the first examiner should carefully record the patient's exact description of the incident. The examiner should not shorten or modify the patient's version of events surrounding the incident in any material way. These initial statements are likely to enter a legal (as well as medical) record, and the impact of misstatements of the patient's recollection can be embarrassing to the physician.

Occasionally, the initial problem will have occurred in the more distant past, and the physician must be more inquisitive to gain the pertinent information. Examples include delayed infection from a gun shot years previously and forgotten use of an implant for bone fixation or joint replacement.

The examiner should be certain to document the patient's immune status, vaccination history, and routine medical history when acquiring initial information.

Physical Examination

Examination of the patient with an FB injury is often highly focused. After determining the patient's history and completing a visual comparison of the affected versus normal extremity, the physician can focus attention on the "injured part." In the case of an injection injury, the examination can be surprisingly benign. In such a case, the physician needs to carefully examine the soft tissue (fascial compartments, tendon sheaths). The key points regarding examination of any injection or FB injury are:

• External appearance: Is a mass visible? Is erythema present? Is coloration equal to normal blood flow?
• Pain: Is the pain localized? Does it vary with motion? Does it describe a normal nerve distribution?
• Palpation: Is there a discrete area of tenderness or firmness or sharpness?
• Range of motion: Is it full? What is the restriction? Is the restriction real or a result of pain?
• Bone alignment or joint stability: Is the skeleton normal?

Changes in sensation or vascular flow can be the result of direct laceration by sharp objects such as glass shards or the result of an indirect dysfunction secondary to concussive force such as would occur from a gun shot wound (GSW) or bullet. Light touch examination and capillary refill are reliable screening methods for most patients.

All proximal lymph nodes should be examined if the FB may be infectious.

USE OF ADDITIONAL INVESTIGATIONAL TOOLS

The most common additional investigational tool is the x-ray. This tool has the advantage of being readily available, affordable, and relatively easy to interpret by all physicians. Aside from readily identifying any associated fractures or joint dislocations, standard radiography can usually detect metallic FBs, many glass objects, and some injection materials. Additionally, x-rays visualize gas within soft tissues, some swelling changes associated with injury, and occasionally, an organic FB that is a density different from the surrounding tissue.

Other tools of potential value in management of FBs include magnetic resonance imaging, computed axial tomography, ultrasound, fluoroscopy, and magnetic resonance angiogram (Table 1).

TREATMENT

Before planning removal of FBs, it should be noted that observing FBs is sometimes the preferred treatment; that is, not all FBs require removal. Gun shot wounds and bullets in particular are good examples of object that can be essentially sterile and not require or benefit from immediate removal. These objects

TABLE 1. *Tools for foreign body management*

	Acute diagnostic value	Direct treatment value	Comments
MRI	High for nonmetal	Low	Consider for localization before exploration
CAT	Probably equaled by radiograph	Very low	Utility surpassed by MRI
Ultrasound	Can identify organic material	Potential utility to find abcess, organic matter	Highly operator dependent, limited availability
Fluroscopy	Clarity poor when compared to other x-ray methods	Very useful for triangulating objects; instruments; known anatomy	Use newer machines with low radiation output or high resolution
MR angiogram	Occasionally useful if vascular injury possible or suspected	Limited	If lesion suspected, plan OR or exploration accordingly

CAT, computed axial tomography; *MR,* magnetic resonance, *MRI,* magnetic resonance imaging; *OR,* operating room.

may be lodged in tight or less accessible places. Unless definite dysfunction or infection is present, the removal of a FB may carry more risk than benefit.

Once the diagnosis of a problematic FB is made and the location of the material has been determined, the physician must choose whether to observe, explore and remove, or explore and débride. One operative certainty is that any wounds and/or incisions should be drained and not closed completely.

Treatment of many FBs can be completed in the ER. This is particularly true regarding FBs within the dorsal aspect of the fingers, pulp tissues, and subcutaneous tissues of the hand and forearm. Critical to the successful removal of FBs in the outpatient or ER arena are:

- Adequate anesthesia or sedation
- Excellent lighting
- Appropriate instruments
- Clean operative field with sterile draping
- Fluoroscopy (This is critical and can save time and reduce pain.)
- Tourniquet availability
- Irrigation
- Connection of individual puncture injuries
- Copious irrigation to clean away the foreign materials
- Often, placement of a drain to promote decompression (particularly if infection is suspected)
- Material collection for appropriate cultures

As a general rule, removal of FBs that are deep to the fascial plane or within the flexor tendon system should be completed in a highly controlled environment. This is particularly true when dealing with foreign agents such as grease, paint, or toxic chemicals. In these cases, the surgeon should be prepared to complete extensive dissections and débridements and, when necessary, apply neutralizing chemicals. In exposure to certain toxic solvents, early débridement and application of counteragents definitely improves outcome.

Many FBs can be managed without hospitalization; however, some patients with FB injuries present to the physician with systemic signs of infection and/or chemical toxicity. For these patients, a period of hospitalization is mandatory. Outpatient administration of antibiotics has made possible the early discharge of these patients once their wound management is stable.

KEY POINTS

The keys to satisfactory outcome are:

• Early identification of infectious agents that are foreign bodies
• Complete decompression of caustic or infectious material
• Early active range of motion of all stable joints and tendons
• Pain management

Patients should be followed closely until wounds have stabilized and any infectious process is resolving. Failure to improve within 24 to 48 hours of any intervention should cause the physician to reexamine the treatment plan.

SELECTED REFERENCES

Anderson MA, Newmeyer WL III, Kilgore ES Jr. Diagnosis and treatment of retained foreign bodies in the hand. Am J Hand Surg 1988;144:63–67.
Boyes JH. Bunnell's surgery of the hand, 5th ed. JB Lippincott, Philadelphia, 1970.
Donaldson JS. Radiographic imaging of foreign bodies in the hand. Hand Clin 1991;7:125–134.
Rayan GM, Putnam JL, Cahill SL, Flournoy DJ. *Eikenella corrodens* in human mouth flora. J Hand Surg 1988;13A:953–956.

34

Complex Regional Pain Syndromes

GENERAL INFORMATION

Arm injuries produce pain. This is not surprising given the density of sensory innervation of the arm. Not only will the patient experience pain from skin incision or laceration, but also from indirect (swelling or traction) and direct (contusion or laceration) of deeper innervated structures, including individual named and unnamed nerves.

Difficulty arises when pain appears greater than that expected from the observed injury. This phenomenon of "pain out of proportion to the observable injury" is often referred to as "complex regional pain syndrome." Unfortunately, this term is imprecise and cannot be universally defined. Some agreement exists that to be considered classic complex regional pain syndrome the patient should exhibit:

1. Pain out of proportion to the provable injury
2. Measurable stiffness of joints in the affected region
3. Observable vasomotor difference in the affected area

DIAGNOSTIC CRITERIA

History

The typical patient with complex regional pain syndrome may not exist; however, some characteristics are seen commonly:

- The patient will likely recall an injury. The injury may not have been severe and no fracture, laceration, or other observable injury may have been noted. The onset of "true complex regional pain syndrome" in the absence of a recalled injury is decidedly uncommon. The physician should detail the recalled injury exactly as the patient states. In work or litigation scenarios, the

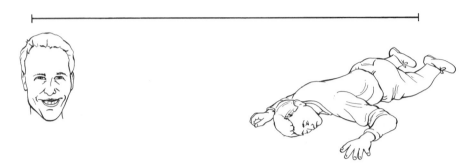

FIG. 1. Visual analog pain scale. The patient is asked to mark the location and volume of the pain. This scale is completed before each visit.

physician should delineate the relation of activity to any aggravation of symptoms.
- The injury may have been "small." Management of the injury is often unremarkable.
- Women develop this condition more often than men.
- This condition rarely occurs in children.

Other factors, such as ongoing addictions (nicotine, prescription drugs, street drugs, ETOH), past history of addictions, involvement in litigation, history of ipsilateral injuries, and current work status should be recorded. No specific past treatment is associated with the onset of complex regional pain syndrome; however, the use of external fixators may have a higher than average rate of pain syndrome development when compared with internal fixation for the same fracture type.

A useful method of assessing the degree of pain experienced by a patient is a visual analog scale (VAS pain scale) (Fig. 1). Having the patient complete this tool after each manipulation assists the physician in assessing the effectiveness of treatments.

Physical Examination

Complex regional pain syndrome can involve one or many joints (Fig. 2). The patient's whole extremity should be examined, beginning with the base of the skull to include the C-spine, shoulder, upper arm, elbow, forearm, wrist, and hand.

Palpation will confirm the preceding visual findings and should not reveal any specific mass, lymph node enlargement, swelling consistent with abscess or cellulitis, or bone or joint instability. Examination of joint motion or stability, tendon, nerve, and vessel function should also be within the range of expected outcome for treatment of a specific injury. Substantial deviation from expected

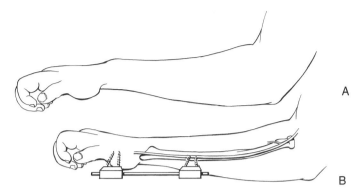

FIG. 2A and B. The patient's hand rests in an "intrinsic minus" position. Different from a more flaccid palsy, the hand is swollen and stiff. The hand could easily be confused with that of a patient who has lost intrinsic muscle function except that, unlike in an intrinsic minus hand, the individual joints are stiff, and the hand is generally swollen. The wrist is slightly flexed, the metacarpophalangeal joints are extended with resultant contracture of the collateral ligaments, and the proximal interphalangeal joints are flexed with associated contracture of the volar plates. Additionally, the hand will be red, warm, and moist or mottled, cool, and shiny and dry. The patient has been treated for an unstable distal radius fracture. Unintentional entrapment of the radial sensory nerve has occurred in conjunction with proximal pin placement.

outcome may indicate that the patient's pain is the result of undertreatment or incomplete treatment of the original injury rather than complex regional pain syndrome (Fig. 2B).

USE OF ADDITIONAL INVESTIGATORY TOOLS

Initial evaluation of any patient with complex regional pain syndrome requires verification of any prior bone or joint reductions and elimination of any concern of underlying infection concern. Usually this can be accomplished with plain x-rays and a complete blood count. The typical patient with complex regional pain syndrome would present similar to the drawing outlined in Fig. 2A, with no untreated pathology, with a normal complete blood count, and an x-ray showing a mottled osteopenia of the carpus (Sudeck's atrophy).

Additional tools of potential value include magnetic resonance imaging, computed axial tomography, Technetium-99 bone scan, electromyogram/nerve conduction velocity testing, and Duplex Doppler vascular flow testing.

Of these testing methods, bone scan screening is often used as a means of identifying those patients whose prior testing has missed key issues. The third or late phase of bone scanning is highly sensitive but poorly specific in identifying the cause of a complex regional pain syndrome. Electromyogram or nerve conduction velocity testing is valuable in identifying those patients with nerve injury or dysfunction who might benefit from additional treatment.

Magnetic resonance imaging, computed axial tomography, and Duplex Doppler testing can be of some value to characterize or diagnose other conditions; however, unlike radionucleotide bone scanning, none of the three is highly sensitive for complex regional pain syndrome.

TREATMENT

The most important issue to consider within differential diagnosis is incomplete treatment or iatrogenic injury. Other diagnoses within the differential include tumors that could reduce vascular outflow from the arm or irritate the brachial plexus. Two examples are lymphoma and Pancoast tumor.

Adson's (1929) efforts to reduce pain by resection of the sympathetic nerve chain were based on the principle of "blocking" the sympathetic pain response. Today, this surgical method has been replaced by the intermittent or repeated administration of sympathetic blocks. Although the method has changed, the principle of reducing sympathetic tone is accepted in combination with therapy and pain medicine management. The goal of treatment should be to break the patient's pain cycle and thereby promote increased motion. Increased motion reduces venous and lymph congestion. Less swelling should further reduce pain and thus lead to even greater motion (Fig. 3). The goals of treatment are to:

• Reduce or control pain
• Increase motion at all "stiff" joints
• Reduce swelling

Tools to manage pain have improved substantially. The physician's toolbox should include narcotic pain medicine, sympathetic blocks, involvement within a pain clinic, and frequent attendance at hand therapy sessions. Although insurers encourage limited use of some of these resources, the treating physician should be a strong advocate for the patient with complex regional pain.

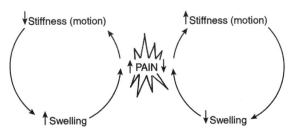

FIG. 3. The presence or absence of pain can affect changes in motion and secondarily swelling, which in turn affects pain.

AFTERCARE

The patient identified with a complex regional pain syndrome requires long-term management. A goal is to educate the patient as to the nature of the diagnosis, the need for home exercises, cessation of aggravating factors, and resolution of any and all confounding issues (litigation, work compensation claims, etc.). To a degree, the patient's result depends on the resolution of these confounding external issues.

EXPECTED OUTCOME

Patients with complex regional pain syndrome are likely to have permanent loss of normal motion in the affected region and chronic cold intolerance. Long-term participation in a pain clinic and therapy program is common. A complete recovery of function is unlikely; however, patients who are discovered during work-up to have treatable causes of pain (partial nerve injury, undiagnosed fractures, etc.) may recover full function depending on the nature of the underlying cause of pain.

The physician's role in maximizing a positive outcome for the patient's is unfamiliar to some. The role shifts from teacher/doer to manager/coordinator. Many physicians do not enjoy interacting with the legal or work compensation system. Successful discharge of a patient correctly diagnosed with complex regional pain syndrome, however, requires that the physician coordinate the maintenance of a pain program and therapy program and simultaneously assist in closure of third-party issues.

MALINGERING

Not all patients diagnosed with complex regional pain syndrome are correctly diagnosed. Separate from patients who are discovered to have other causes for complex pain during their medical work-up are patients who have not been found to have definite diagnoses other than complex regional pain syndrome. Close inspection reveals that they do not have joint stiffness and/or a visible disturbance of vasomotor balance. When such a patient also has no supporting radiographic or radionucleotide evidence, the diagnosis of complex regional pain syndrome should be called into question. This chapter is not intended to fully review the issue of malingering or secondary gain; however, the physician should be aware of the following "red flags":

- Patients who do not appear concerned over their reported pain or loss of function
- Patients who cannot gain "any" relief from their pain
- Patients who begin every visit focused on issues external to their medical care
- Patients who do not have measurable stiffness in the painful area despite complaints of severe pain

If the treating physician is uncertain regarding the validity of the patient's pain, a referral to the psychologist or psychiatrist should be suggested. The patient's response to this referral can be telling. Patients who desire to recover should welcome any and all medical care suggested by their physician; whereas patients concerned about being discovered may balk or refuse to participate in such an evaluation.

SELECTED REFERENCES

Adson AW, Brown GE. Raynaud's disease of the upper extremities: successful treatment by resection of sympathetic cervicothoracic and second thoracic ganglions and intervening truck. JAMA 1929;92:444.

Amadio PC, Mackinnon SE, Merrit WH, Brody GS, Tersis JK. Reflex sympathetic dystrophy syndrome: consensus report of an ad hoc committee of the American Association for Hand Surgery on the definition of reflex sympathetic dystrophy syndrome. J Plast Reconstr Surg 1991;87:371–375.

Mackinnon SE, Holder LE. The use of three-phase radionuclide in the diagnosis of reflex sympathetic dystrophy. J Hand Surg 1984;9A:556.

Watson HK, Carlson L. Treatment of reflex dystrophy of the hand with an active "stress loading" program. J Hand Surg 1987;12A:779.

35

Clenched Fist Syndrome, Factitious Limb Edema, and Self-Inflicted Injury

GENERAL INFORMATION

Occasionally, primary psychiatric diseases manifest as fixed, dramatically abnormal hand postures, factitious limb edema, and self-inflicted injury. These patients truly believe a major condition exists and become upset and indignant if these beliefs are called into question.

DIAGNOSTIC CRITERIA

History

Patients usually present evaluation of fixed digital flexion that occurred spontaneously or following a trivial injury. The patient states that the fingers will not straighten. Although any hand posture is possible, most often patients describe the fingers as fixed in the position of a clenched fist.

Physical Examination

Patients have normal extensor creases. Passive digital extension is associated with significant pain. Typically, the patient holds the long ring and small fingers rigidly flexed, while maintaining normal thumb and index finger mobility. Attempts to straighten the finger actively cause severe pain. If the patient is able to straighten his fingers, attempts at measuring grip are met with "breakaway" resistance. The patient may resist finger extension initially, then suddenly relax and cry out in pain.

Patients with this disorder may deliberately alter the appearance of the hand.

Circumferential edema of the hand or wrist with a discrete proximal margin is a cardinal sign of nonphysiologic disorders. Other patients will repeatedly strike their hand against an object, creating a hard edema on the dorsum of the hand often termed Secrétan's edema. Finally, patients may inflict wounds on themselves and present with chronic nonhealing ulcers.

TREATMENT

Factitious hand disorders are diagnoses of exclusion. These conditions should be considered in patients with a history and physical examination that do not make sense. If a psychiatric condition is suspected, one should refer the patient to a psychiatrist. Patients with self-inflicted lacerations should be treated with local care and casting to protect the site of injury. Patients with a clenched fist or other posturing disorder of the hand may require general anesthesia to correctly diagnose the abnormal hand position. Often the patient will benefit from short periods of casting in a safe position to avoid injury to the skin. The patients underlying psychological condition must be treated for these conditions to improve. Surgical treatment is not indicated.

KEY POINTS

• Factitious disorders present with unusual hand postures or appearances.
• The diagnosis is one of exclusion and evaluation for other disorders is necessary.
• Treatment addresses the psychiatric abnormality.

SELECTED REFERENCES

Grunert BK, et al. Classification system for factitious syndromes in the hand with implications for treatment. J Hand Surg 1991;16A:1027–1030.
Louis DL, et al. The upper extremity and psychiatric illness. J Hand Surg 1985;10A:687–693.
Walle PE, et al. The S-H-A-F-T syndrome in the upper extremity. J Hand Surg 1978;5:492–494.

36

Emergency Room Assessment

Injuries of the hand are one of the more common reasons patients seek emergency department evaluation. Hand injuries may be isolated or part of multiple trauma. Small lacerations, limited blunt trauma, or crush injuries can cause major compromise to hand function. A systematic, detailed examination of the entire arm is important in the hand-injured patient and must not be overlooked in multitrauma patients.

PATIENTS WITH UNSTABLE CONDITIONS

As in many emergency room (ER) situations, formal assessment begins with observation of heart rate, respiration, blood pressure, and temperature. Open injuries and blunt trauma with apparent blood loss or any hypotensive episode are treated with prompt fluid resuscitation using the infusion of 1 to 2 L of intravenous (IV) lactated Ringer's solution. Profound hypotension in the setting of substantial blood loss is emergently treated with non–cross-matched O-negative blood transfusions. Whenever possible, cross-matched, type-specific blood is transfused as time and availability permits. Substantial hypotension resulting from blood loss following hand or upper extremity injuries may indicate a major arterial injury. In this situation, the first maneuver is direct pressure applied just proximal to the site of suspected arterial injury. Alternatively, a blood pressure cuff or surgical tourniquet can be applied and elevated to 250 mm Hg. The use of these methods should be temporary. Definitive treatment should be undertaken promptly by the appropriate consulting service. The use of makeshift tourniquets is discouraged because high edge pressures can cause significant additional soft-tissue injury. Patients with major arterial injury need urgent operative evaluation. A brief history and examination are obtained as time permits. The salient points of the history are obtained from relatives if the patient is not communicative. The injured extremity is splinted and a compressive dressing applied. The early application of a splint aides in blood loss and pain control.

PATIENTS WITH STABLE CONDITIONS

History

The formal ER assessment then continues with a survey of the history of present illness, past medical history, and review of systems. The evaluating physician should first identify the patient's age, handedness, and occupation. The history of present illness should focus on the circumstances surrounding the incident, including time of injury of onset of symptoms, nature of the injury, as well as the patient's functional and pain complaints. If the injury was caused by a piece of machinery, the specifications of the machine (such as revolutions per minute or pounds of torque produced) may help further define the injury. Injuries occurring while on the job should be so noted in the medical record. In addition to such pertinent factors as major illness, medications, last tetanus immunization, previous fractures, or surgery of the injured limb, smoking history should also be queried. If surgery is anticipated, the time of the patient's last oral intake should be determined. (See Chapter 3, History, for a further discussion of the evaluation of hand injuries.)

Physical Examination

Next, in order to examine the hand, any initially applied splint or dressing is removed. In some extenuating circumstances, the surgeon may not examine the extremity until the patient has been transferred to the operating room. A systematic examination of the hand and arm is performed, focusing on the condition of the integument, neurologic condition (sensory and motor function), individual tendon function, vascular status, edema, gross alignment of the extremity, and skeletal integrity. Ecchymosis, deformity, or length of lacerations or skin defects should be noted in the medical record. Performing an Allen's test can assess differential patency of the radial and ulnar arteries. A focused neurologic examination should be accomplished, assessing the motor function of the ulnar, median, and radial nerves independently. Any penetrating wound overlying the radial or ulnar artery should be suspected of involving that artery. Recent data advises to the contrary, it is better to rely on an exam. In most situations it is preferable to refrain from delivering systemic pain medications or local anesthesia until a full examination is completed. The injured extremity is always inspected with comparison made to the contralateral side. Any energy imparted to the hand and wrist region, whether resulting in a laceration or contusion, can cause a fracture or dislocation. Based on the patient's initial survey (and once the patient is stabilized), blunt or penetrating injuries must have orthogonal, 90-degree biplanar x-rays of the appropriate body part (Table 1). If appropriate, it is preferable to obtain biplanar x-rays out of any splints applied in the field. It is also preferable that the biplanar x-rays are obtained by moving the radiographic beam and not the extremity. The consulting surgeon should be contacted if questions arise regarding appropriateness of splint removal or positioning.

TABLE 1. *Radiographic for blunt or penetrating injuries*

Isolated digital trauma	PA, lateral, and oblique
Hand trauma	PA, lateral, and oblique
Wrist trauma	PA and lateral[a]
Forearm trauma	AP and lateral
Elbow trauma	AP and lateral

[a]Obtaining the PA wrist film in neutral forearm rotation is critically important. This is done by positioning the shoulder at 90 degrees abduction with the wrist placed flat on the x-ray cassette. The x-ray beam is directed from a posterior to anterior direction. For further reference, see Chapter 4, Physical Examination of the Hand.

AP, anterior posterior; *PA,* posterior anterior.

Laceration should be thoroughly inspected and probed to identify full thickness penetration. Suspicion should be high for tendon laceration in the setting of full thickness skin penetration on either the volar or dorsal aspect of the hand and forearm. The digital extensor and flexor tendons must be individually assessed for injury. If the patient can offer digital resistance but complains of pain during the examination of any tendon, the examiner should consider the presence of partial tendon laceration. (See Chapter 14, Soft-Tissue Injuries and Lacerations; Chapter 15, Extensor Tendon Injuries; and Chapter 16, Flexor Tendon Injuries.)

Initial Treatment

After the initial physical examination is complete and an appropriate surgical or procedural consent has been obtained, oral, IV, or intramuscular (IM) pain medication may be administered for patient comfort. Local anesthesia can be useful if hand wounds are to be explored or repaired. This is typically obtained with the injection of 1% lidocaine without epinephrine. The digital block is a useful anesthetic tool for repair of nail injuries, repair of simple digital extensor mechanism injuries, exploration of lacerations, laceration repair, and fracture or dislocation reduction (Chapter 6, Anesthesia for Hand Surgery).

A custom-applied well-padded plaster or fiberglass splint is applied for patient comfort and to prevent any progression of injury. A liberal amount of padding is applied, particularly about the bony prominences. If plaster is used, 10 sheets of 5- × 30-inch material are dipped in warm water for 10 to 15 seconds, then applied to the hand, wrist, and forearm. Simply conforming the plaster about the digits in an extended position is acceptable and may actually aid in edema control because this splintage is temporary. The splint is secured by the application of a nonconstricting bandage such as a lightly applied elastic wrap. Care must be exercised to not apply the Ace wrap too tightly. It is of paramount importance to strictly elevate the extremity above the level of the heart and apply an ice pack following the initial ER assessment of the hand injury and while awaiting definitive management. Such antiedema maneuvers facilitate ultimate management of the hand, wrist, or forearm injury.

Consultations with appropriate surgical subspecialists are often necessary for the multitrauma patient. In preparation for surgery, general medical evaluation is necessary in patients with complicated medical conditions. Although tedious, clear, organized, and accurate ER records are essential for continuity of care and medical–legal defense. Additionally, written notes can be supplemented with drawing of wounds and lacerations.

SELECTED REFERENCES

Aulicino PL. Clinical examination of the hand. In: Hunter JM, Mackin EJ, Callahan AD, eds. Rehabilitation of the hand: surgery and therapy. Mosby, St. Louis, 1995, pp. 53–75.

Cooney WP, Bishop AT, Linscheid RL. Physical examination of the wrist. In: Cooney WP, ed. The wrist: diagnosis and operative treatment. Mosby, St. Louis, pp. 236–261.

Harkess JW, Ramsey WC, Harkess JW. Principles of fractures and dislocations. In: Rockwood CA, Green DP, Bucholz RW, Heckman JD, eds. Fractures in adults, 4th ed. Lippincott-Raven, Philadelphia, pp. 3–120.

Hoppenfeld SL. Examination of the extremities. Appleton and Lange, Norwalk, Connecticut, 1976.

Smith KL. Wound care for the hand patient. In: Hunter JM, Mackin EJ, Callahan AD, eds. Rehabilitation of the hand: surgery and therapy. Mosby, St. Louis, pp. 237–250.

The hand: physical examination and diagnosis. American Society for Surgery of the Hand, Chicago, 1992.

37

The Operating Room in Hand Surgery

GENERAL INFORMATION

The operating room setup for hand surgery is unique among the surgical disciplines. Surgical retractors and other instruments used in general orthopedic surgery are too large and of little use in hand surgery. It is important for the operating room technicians and nurses to have special instrument trays available for hand surgery (Table 1). It is also important for the operating room surgeon to realize that the uniqueness of hand surgery instruments may result in some surgical support staff being unfamiliar with their use. Instrument room personnel must be reminded of the fine caliber of hand surgery instruments, taking special care not to bend or otherwise damage them during processing. The operating surgeons must also exercise care in handling these instruments. Positioning of the patient on the operating room table as well as anesthetic alternatives deserve special consideration in hand surgery.

PATIENT POSITIONING, PREPARATION, AND OPERATING ROOM SETUP

For the majority of hand surgical procedures, the patient is positioned supine on an operating room table with the operated hand placed on a hand surgery table that is stabilized with two legs. This table is well padded to prevent pressure sores or contusion to the ulnar nerve. The table is constructed of a radiolucent material, such as Plexiglas or wood, to enable radiographic examination of the hand. Once the patient is positioned, the surgeon should ensure that the contralateral elbow and wrist are well padded and positioned free from pressure or irritation. Likewise, padding is placed beneath the knees and heels to prevent pressure injury that might occur during a prolonged procedure. The knees are positioned in a slightly flexed position to prevent injury to the perineal nerve. Because of the rich vascularity of the hand and upper extremity, procedures are typically performed under a tourniquet. A well-padded 18-inch pneumatic

TABLE 1. *Contents of standard hand surgery instrument tray*

Army Navy retractor	Straight and curved mosquito forceps
Mallet	Kelly clamps
Angled ronguer	Allis clamps
Straight ronguer	Right angle clamps
Small pliers	Scalpel handles
Weitlander retractors	Beaver blade handles
Osteotomes	Adson forceps
Small curettes	Nerve hook
Mayo needle holder	Freer elevator
Tenotomy scissors	Small rasp
Straight and curved Mayo scissors	$1/4$" Key elevator
Towel clamps	Single and double skin hooks
Littler scissors	

tourniquet is applied to the upper arm for most surgical procedures. Some prefer the use of a forearm or wrist tourniquet for certain procedures. Of particular importance is to ensure that the edges of the tourniquet have been sufficiently padded prior to tourniquet inflation. Skin injury following tourniquet usage is most frequently seen beneath the tourniquet edge. Care is taken to place an impervious barrier just distal to the tourniquet to prevent the seepage of solutions beneath the tourniquet during the preparing and draping of the extremity. The extremity can be scrubbed with a variety of solutions, including a combination of Hibiclens, alcohol, or Betadine. Sustained scrubbing for 7 to 10 minutes is sufficient. At the conclusion of the surgical scrub and prior to draping, some surgeons prefer to paint the exposed limb with Betadine. The arm can be draped using commercially available hand drapes that generously cover the patient while also accommodating the hand table.

The surgeon is seated at the hand table, most commonly facing the medial aspect of the arm, also known as the "axilla side" of the patient. The first assistant sits facing the surgeon and the surgical technician is seated at the end of the

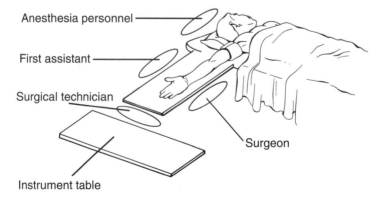

FIG. 1. Operating room setup.

hand table. A separate instrument table is positioned immediately within reach of the surgical technician and surgeon (Fig. 1). Some surgeons find sitting on the opposite side of the arm easier for operations that involve the dorsum of the hand or wrist.

STERILE TECHNIQUE

A surgical mask, head cover, foot covers, and scrubs must be donned prior to entering the operating room. As in all surgical procedures, sterile technique must be observed at all times. The surgeon or surgical assistant performs a 5- to 7-minute brush scrub before gowning and gloving. The scrub can be accomplished with either Hibiclens or Betadine solution. Once the scrub is completed, the surgeon opens the operating room door with his or her back and then proceeds directly to the gowned surgical assistant, who will then, in turn, assist him or her in gowning. Until gowned and gloved, the surgeon should never pass directly between the draped patient and the sterile instrument table. Once gowned, the surgeon should never pass in proximity to an assistant's or technician's unsterile back. Surgeons should only pass "front to front." The use of cloth or paper gowns vary from hospital to hospital but the surgeon or surgical assistant should request a generous gown size, because once seated these gowns may "creep up" exposing unsterile areas of the legs or lap region. Glove sizes should not be tight because this can cause pain and fatigue during lengthy surgeries. Double gloving is recommended in order to minimize the risk of blood-borne diseases.

It is important for the surgeon and assistant to remember that breaks in sterility can occur more easily when they are seated. When arising from the seated position, the surgeon and assistant must exercise caution in preventing the "lap area" from coming into contact with the operating field. Another common break in sterility during hand surgery occurs when the surgeon or assistant arises from a seated position, contaminating the surgical light handle with the top of the head. Although tempting, the surgeon should not recover and reuse instruments that have dropped into the surgeon or assistant's lap.

ANESTHESIA

Choices available for hand surgery anesthesia include general, regional, or local. The anesthesiologist, based on the patient's general health, typically makes the choice of anesthesia. Procedures requiring one or more surgical sites, such as anterior iliac crest bone graft harvest for scaphoid nonunion reconstruction, necessitate a general inhalation anesthetic. The use of regional anesthesia, such as an axillary block, is extremely useful in hand surgery. Not only does it obviate the need for a general anesthetic, but also it can provide prolonged postoperative pain relief (sometimes up to 12 hours). For brief surgical procedures, such as carpal tunnel release or trigger finger release, local anesthesia with or without the use of conscious intravenous sedation is used. Local anesthesia is commonly performed by the surgeon, using small amounts of 1% lidocaine, without epinephrine, delivered through a small-gauge (25-gauge) needle.

TOURNIQUET

The arm is exsanguinated with an elastic bandage prior to surgical incision and after the final surgical plan is made. For adults, the tourniquet is usually inflated to 250 mm Hg. In children and adolescents, the tourniquet pressure should be set 100 mm Hg above the systolic blood pressure. Prolonged ischemia is obviously a potentially hazardous situation. Muscle histologic changes have been shown during the course of tourniquet with the pH of the arm musculature dropping to 6.9 following 2 hours of tourniquet usage; therefore, the tourniquet should be inflated for no more than 2 hours. For prolonged procedures, the tourniquet can be deflated for 20 minutes to allow limb reperfusion prior to reinflation.

INSTRUMENTATION

Small precision instruments are required for successful hand surgery. The hand surgical instrument tray should include the fine forceps also known as Adson forceps. Long- and short-handled tenotomy scissors are needed for dissection about the hand, wrist, and forearm. These scissors may become bent or dull, requiring periodic repair or replacement. Number 15- and 11-blade scalpels are used frequently for skin incisions as well as deeper dissection. More delicate sharp dissection is sometimes accomplished with a no. 69 Beaver blade. At least two knives should be on each surgical setup to prevent unnecessary downtime incurred while changing scalpel blades. A variety of retractors are available for hand surgery and usage often depends on the surgeon's preference. Versatile and popular retractors include single- and double-pronged hooks, Senn retractors, and Ragnell retractors. The availability of these instruments provides the surgeon with the option of sharp or blunt surfaces for retraction. Self-retaining retractors are also useful.

It is advisable for most hand surgery procedures to be performed with the aid of magnification, preferably 2× or 3.5× enhancement. Ideally, this is done using custom-made glasses with focal length appropriate for a seated surgeon focusing on a hand table.

SELECTED REFERENCES

Green DP. General principles. In: Green DP, ed. Green's operative hand surgery, 4th ed. Churchill Livingstone, New York, 1998, pp. 1–20.

Harkess JW, Ramsey WC, Harkess JW. Principles of fractures and dislocations. In: Rockwood CA, Green DP, Bucholz RW, Heckman JD, eds. Fractures in adults, 4th ed. Lippincott-Raven, Philadelphia, 1997, pp. 3–120.

Milford L. Surgical technique and aftercare. In: Crenshaw AH, ed. Campbell's operative orthopaedics, 7th ed. Mosby, St. Louis, 1987, pp. 111–137.

Smith KL. Wound care for the hand patient. In: Hunter JM, Mackin EJ, Callahan AD, eds. Rehabilitation of the hand: surgery and therapy. Mosby, St. Louis, 1995, pp. 237–250.

38

Aftercare of the Injured and Operated Hand

GENERAL INFORMATION

Appropriate aftercare is critical to a successful result following hand injuries or elective hand surgery. Following injury or operation, specific splints or casts are necessary in most situations. Rehabilitation protocols administered by a certified hand therapist are paramount to the recovery of patients with hand injuries or for patients recovering from hand surgery. Disregard for the principles of hand immobilization and hand rehabilitation is one of the single greatest contributing factors to poor outcome from hand surgery or injury. In general, hand surgery is a discipline that frequently employs motion. Treatment of hand conditions has as its primary goal early motion. Dressing, splints, and rehabilitation protocols should facilitate this goal.

WOUND DRESSING AND EDEMA CONTROL

Postoperative dressings for the hand and wrist should be nonadherent and nonconstrictive. A moist wound covering such as Adaptic or Zeroform should be applied to the wound, followed by dry gauze sponges. A forgiving circular dressing such as soft-roll or Webril is used to stabilize the sponges. The preferred outer wrap is stockinet cut on the bias. Alternatively "ace-wraps" can be used as a hand and arm dressing but care must be exercised during application because of a tendency by many to stretch this elastic bandage too tightly, causing a constrictive dressing. If a digital dressing is to be applied, a small 2 × 2 inch gauze applied with a lightly applied, single-layer 2-in. Kling, secured with a top dressing of 1/2-in. Coban may be used. If motion is to be encouraged after the application of hand, wrist, or digital dressing, the dressing should not be thick and multilayered but lightly applied particularly about the joint creases. Sustained hand elevation with application of ice is encouraged to decrease postoperative or postinjury edema. This can be facilitated by using commercially available arm elevators or by propping the extremity above the heart using pillows (Fig. 1).

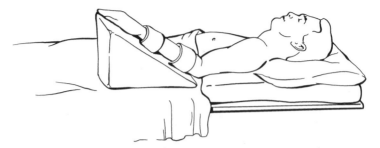

FIG. 1. Arm elevation.

HAND POSITION

The safe position of immobilization of the proximal interphalangeal joint (PIP) is approximately 30 degrees of flexion, because this puts the collateral ligaments of the PIP joint on their greatest tension. Theoretically, therefore, the ligaments should not be subject to contracture following a period of immobilization and prolonged PIP stiffness should not result. Similarly, the metacarpophalangeal (MCP) joint is protected from contracture when it is immobilized in 90 degrees of flexion. This places the collateral ligaments on maximum tension because of the "cam effect" of the MCP. The shape of the metacarpal head is oval such that, when the MCP is held in extension, the collateral ligaments are lax, and they are taught when the MCP is held in maximum flexion (Fig. 2). Immobilizing the MCP in maximum flexion prohibits post-

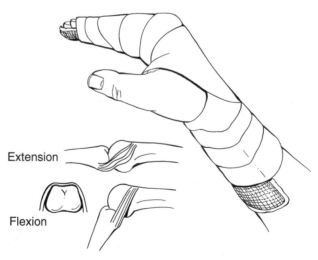

Extension

Flexion

FIG. 2. Safe position. *Inset* shows tension applied to the collateral ligaments with the MCP joint in the "safe position."

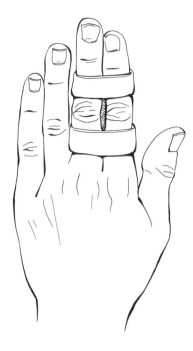

FIG. 3. Buddy taping.

splinting stiffness of the MCP. The "prehensile position of the wrist" or the position of function of the wrist is approximately 15 degrees of extension. Prolonged positioning of the wrist in flexion promotes stiffness of the digits by promoting contracture of the intrinsic musculature. The wrist has a wide range of motion in flexion and extension and it is more desirable to sacrifice wrist flexion than wrist extension because most hand activities depend on wrist extension. As a general rule for immobilization in the upper extremity, joints above and below the area in question should be immobilized.

For nondisplaced or minimally displaced phalangeal fractures, early digital motion can be started using the immobilization technique of "buddy taping." Buddy taping is accomplished by placing a small piece of gauze between the PIP joint prominences of adjacent digits then securing them by tape applied about the fingers at the level of the proximal phalanges and the level of the middle phalanges (Fig. 3). Care is taken to not restrict the motion of the MCP, PIP, or distal interphalangeal joint.

MONITORING

Medical support personnel or the patient's family must monitor the hand following treatment of hand injuries. The hand should be monitored for adequacy of arterial inflow, adequacy of venous outflow, and integrity of nerve function.

Even in the confines of a splint, the motor and sensory function of the median, ulnar, and radial nerves usually can be specifically assessed.

GENERAL RULES OF HAND THERAPY

The most important goals following hand surgery or treatment from a hand injury are early mobilization and edema control; therefore, following surgical intervention or nonoperative injury treatment, the patient is encouraged to initiate such exercises as "overhead fisting." With rare exception, this exercise can be done without risk of compromising the treatment course. In accomplishing this exercise, the patient flexes the shoulder above the head and pumps the fist. This accentuates digital venous and lymphatic return as well as preventing shoulder stiffness (adhesive capsulitis). Elbow range of motion is also encouraged, preferably above shoulder level to prevent dependent edema.

With injuries at the wrist or above, digital motion is also strongly encouraged by instructing the patient on active and passive range of motion, including isolated finger joint techniques. The patient concentrates on the motion of specific joints while restricting the movement of adjacent joints. Further hand therapy can be accomplished by patient referral to a certified hand therapist for instruction on "six-pack" hand exercises, which are a group of universally employed digital mobilization maneuvers. Edema is also controlled by the application of individual digital wraps using Coban in the same fashion as the ace-wrap is applied to the extremity. The use of "buddy taping" techniques can encourage motion in stiff digits by attaching them to digits with full active range of motion.

HAND THERAPY FOR SPECIFIC CONDITIONS

Flexor Tendon Injuries

The most challenging and unique area of hand rehabilitation is that of digital flexor tendon injuries. Specific protocols have been developed for these injuries. These protocols focus on early mobilization and have been created based on the strength of the suturing technique. As flexor tendon repairs have become stronger, the immediate passive motion and early active motion protocols have become more widely used. The strength of the flexor tendon repair is based on the number of sutures passed through the repair site. The most popular type of flexor tendon repair is one that places four sutures across the tendon repair site. This is known as the "four-strand" repair. Mobilization of flexor tendon repair generally commences no later than postoperative day 5. A custom molded Orthoplast splint is fashioned with the wrist is 15 degrees of flexion and 70 to 90 degrees MCP joint flexion. Within the confines of the splint, passive range of motion exercises are initiated. Additionally, "place and hold" exercises are initiated in most circumstances. By the third postoperative week, the patient is instructed on early active range of motion within the splint and wrist "tenodesis" motion out of the splint is begun. Splinting is discontinued by postoperative week 6.

Alternatively, a dynamic flexion splint may be worn for 6 weeks, which allows immediate active extension while permitting passive digital flexion through the action of rubber band outriggers originating from the flexor surface of the splint. This splint is commonly referred to as the "Kleinert" apparatus.

Extensor Tendon Injuries

The cornerstone of multiple extensor tendon repair rehabilitation is the concept of active digital flexion and passive digital extension. This is facilitated by the use of a dynamic extension outrigger splint with outriggers originating from the extensor surface of the forearm. This device is commonly removed between postoperative weeks 4 and 6. Isolated extensor tendon injuries or some multiple extensor tendon injuries below the level of the wrist may be rehabilitated without the need of dynamic extension outrigger splints.

General Fracture Care

Fractures of the digits can be treated with splint immobilization, percutaneous pinning, buddy taping, or internal fixation. Splinting techniques and percutaneous pinning techniques require a period of initial immobilization ranging from 3 to 4 weeks in most circumstances. After removal of the splint or the percutaneous pins, active and passive mobilization can begin under the supervision of a hand therapist. With the use of buddy tape stabilization or internal fixation, immediate active and gentle passive motion is accomplished in most settings. Exceptions to this may include the complex reconstruction of intraarticular fractures or fractures with radiographic signs of delayed union. Once range of motion is initiated, patients are generally given a custom molded resting splint for protection.

Reflex Sympathetic Dystrophy (Sympathetic Mediated Pain Syndrome)

Complex or simple injuries of the hand or the digits can be complicated by the "shoulder hand arm syndrome," also known as reflex sympathetic dystrophy (RSD). In this condition, a sympathetically mediated condition may cause stiffness, edema, and pain in the digits as well as the wrist, elbow, and shoulder. Diagnosed early, this condition responds to aggressive active and passive range of motion therapy. Prophylactic mobilization and "desensitization" of the entire upper extremity may prevent this condition. Nerve blocks of the stellate ganglion, however, are often necessary.

The Poorly Motivated Patient

Unfortunately, some patients may not grasp the serious nature of hand injuries or the importance that hand therapy plays in regaining use of their injured extremity. In these circumstances, the surgeon and therapist must realize the importance of frequent follow-up of the patient's progress. In these situations, the hand therapist plays a pivotal role by being the surgeon's "eyes" and "ears" as well as the person who is "hands on" with the patient. Certain patients need pushing, encouragement, and reeducation on a frequent basis in order to achieve postoperative goals. Although not necessarily "poorly motivated," some patients become extremely apprehensive and leery of rehabilitation, often because of fear. Hand therapy can play a vital role in restoring patient confidence, thereby further facilitating recovery.

MODALITIES

Depending on the state, occupational therapists, physical therapists, or both may deliver "treatment modalities" to hand surgery patients. These commonly include ultrasound phonophoresis, iontophoresis, transelectrical stimulation (TENS) unit, fluidotherapy, electrical stimulation, paraffin treatments, and heat contrast baths. Phonophoresis utilizes 10% hydrocortisone cream and is typically delivered with an ultrasound probe directly to the area of concern. The TENS unit uses a small, steady battery-generated current to desensitize patients to chronic pain. TENS unit stimulate large myelinated nerve fibers thereby closing the gates for further pain transmission. Using the principal of ionizing current, iontophoresis infiltrates soft tissues with hydrocortisone cream, directly over the area of concern. Fluidotherapy is delivered with a device that places the hand in indirect contact to circulating particles. These particles striking the hand more or less act as a "deep massage" and may aid in mobilization of the digits. Contrast baths may decrease edema, diminish pain, and augment digital motion. Patients may learn the technique of contrast bathing for their hands, using the modality at home. Paraffin "dressings" may be applied under the direction of a therapist, aiding in digital mobilization and edema control. Generally not considered a pain relieving modality, electrical stimulation is used to help gain digital motion by direct stimulation to the specific muscle or muscles controlling the digit in question.

SELECTED REFERENCES

Evan RB, McAuliffe JA. Wound class and management. In: Hunter JM, Mackin EJ, Callahan AD, eds. Rehabilitation of the hand: surgery and therapy. Mosby, St. Louis, 1995, pp. 217–236.

Harkess JW, Ramsey WC, Harkess JW. Principles of fractures and dislocations. In: Rockwood CA, Green DP, Bucholz RW, Heckman JD, eds. Fractures in adults, 4th ed. Lippincott-Raven, Philadelphia, 1997, pp. 3–120.

Milford L. Surgical technique and aftercare. In: Crenshaw AH, ed. Campbell's operative orthopaedics. Mosby, St. Louis, 1987, pp. 111–137.

Smith KL. Wound care for the hand patient. In: Hunter JM, Mackin EJ, Callahan AD, eds. Rehabilitation of the hand: surgery and therapy. Mosby, St. Louis, 1995, pp. 237–250.

Suggested Readings

Anderson JE. Grant's atlas of anatomy, 7th ed. Williams & Wilkins, Baltimore, 1978.

Buck-Gramcko D, ed. Congenital malformations of the hand and forearm. Churchill Livingstone, London, 1998.

Chase RA. Atlas of hand surgery. WB Saunders, Philadelphia, 1973.

Cooney WP, Linscheid RL, Dobyns JH, eds. The wrist: diagnosis and operative treatment. Mosby, St. Louis, 1998.

Freeland AE. Hand fractures. Repair, reconstruction and rehabilitation. Churchill Livingstone, Philadelphia, 2000.

Gelberman RH. Operative nerve repair & reconstruction. JB Lippincott, Philadelphia, 1991.

Green DP, Hotchkiss RN, Pederson WC. Green's operative hand surgery, 4th ed. Churchill Livingstone, New York, 1999.

Henry A. Extensile exposure, 2nd ed. Churchill Livingstone, London, 1973.

Hollinshead WH. Anatomy for surgeons, vol. 3, 3rd ed. Harper & Row, Philadelphia, 1982.

Hunter JM, Schneider LH, Mackin EJ, Callahan AD. Rehabilitation of the hand, 4th ed. Mosby, St. Louis, 1995.

Kaplan E. Functional and surgical anatomy of the hand, 2nd ed. JB Lippincott, Philadelphia, 1965.

Lampe EW. Surgical anatomy of the hand. CIBA Clin Symp 1988;40:1.

Mann RJ. Infections of the hand. Lea & Febiger, Philadelphia, 1988.

Peimer CA. Surgery of the hand and upper extremity, vol. 1 and 2. McGraw-Hill, New York, 1966.

Spinner M. Injuries to the major branches of peripheral nerves of the forearm, 2nd ed. WB Saunders, Philadelphia, 1978.

Spinner M. Kaplan's functional and surgical anatomy of the hand, 3rd ed. JB Lippincott, Philadelphia, 1984.

Trumble T. Principles of hand surgery & therapy. WB Saunders, Philadelphia, 2000.

Appendix 1

Key to Abbreviations

ADM	Abductor digit minimi		FDM	Flexor digit minimi
AdP	Adductor pollicis		FDP	Flexor digitorum profundus
APB	Abductor pollicis brevis		FDS	Flexor digitorum superficialis
APL	Abductor pollicis longus		FPB	Flexor pollicis brevis
CMC	Carpometacarpal		FPL	Flexor pollicis longus
DIP	Distal interphalangeal joint		HPII	High pressure injection injury
ECRB	Extensor carpi radialis brevis		I	Index finger
ECRL	Extensor carpi radialis longus		IP	Interphalangeal
ECU	Extensor carpi ulnaris		M	Middle finger
EDC	Extensor digitorum communis		MCP	Metacarpophalangeal
EDM	Extensor digiti minimi		ODM	Opponens digiti minimi
EIP	Extensor indicis proprius		OP	Opponens pollicis
EPB	Extensor pollicis brevis		PIP	Proximal interphalangeal
EPL	Extensor pollicis longus		PL	Palmaris longus
FB	Foreign body		R	Ring finger
FCR	Flexor carpi radialis		S	Small finger
FCU	Flexor carpi ulnaris			

Appendix 2

Anatomy: Summary

Joint control	Prime muscle[a]	Nerve	Figure number	Comments
Wrist				
Flexion	Flexor carpi radialis	Median		Absence, weak wrist
	Palmaris longus	Median		Flexion present by flexor digitorum
	Flexor carpi ulnaris	Ulnar		superficialis, flexor digitorum profundus
Extension	Extensor carpi radialis longus			Absence, wrist drop
Radial	Extensor carpi radialis longus	Radial		
Ulnar	Extensor carpi ulnaris	Radial		
Finger metacarpophalangeal				
Flexion	Interosseous	Ulnar	1	Absence, claw hand
Extension	Extensor digitorum communis		2. Also see physical exam, figs. 7 and 8	Absence, metacarpophalangeal extensor lag
Abduction	Dorsal	Ulnar	See physical exams 12 and 13	
Adduction	Volar	Ulnar		
Finger proximal interphalangeal				
Flexion	Flexor digitorum superficialis	Median	See physical exam 3	Must block flexor digitorum profundus to detect clinical absence
Extension	Interosseous	Ulnar		Intrinsic independent of metacarpophalangeal position: extrinsic only if metacarpophalangeal Joint flexed or at 0 degrees (i.e., not hyperextended)

(continued)

253

Joint control	Prime muscle[a]	Nerve	Figure number	Comments
Finger distal interphalangeal				
Flexion	Flexor digitorum profundus	Median, index and middle fingers Ulnar ring little	See physical exam 2	
Extension	None			Strong distal interphalangeal extension contingent on active proximal interphalangeal extension control
Thumb CMCJ				
Flexion	Flexor pollicis brevis			
Extension	Abductor pollicis longus			
Opposition	Abductor pollicis brevis	Median		A composite motion
Supination	Extensor pollicis longus	Radial		
Thumb metacarpophalangeal				
Flexion	Flexor pollicis longus	Median		
Thumb interphalangeal				
Flexion	Flexor pollicis longus	Median	See physical exam 1	
Extension	Extension pollicis longus	Radial		Weak interphalangeal extension Also by intrinsics

[a]Achieves a given function but does not imply the strongest acting across that joint.

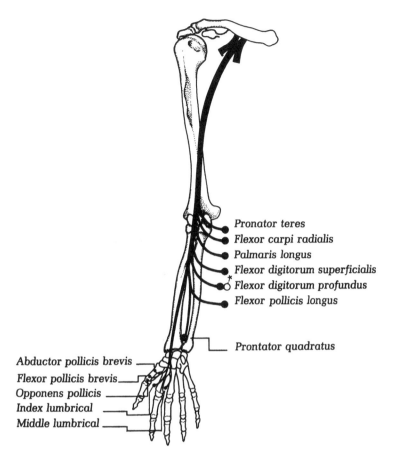

FIG. 1. Median and anterior interosseus nerves. Muscles innervated by the median and anterior interosseous nerves in the forearm and hand.

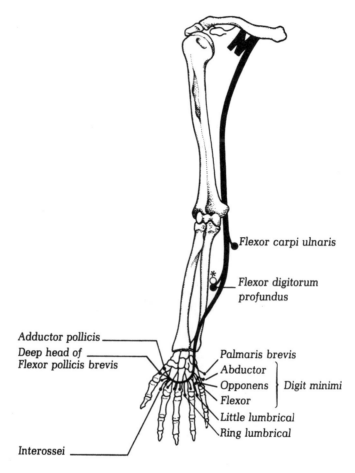

FIG. 2. Ulnar nerve. Muscles innervated by the ulnar nerve in the forearm and hand.

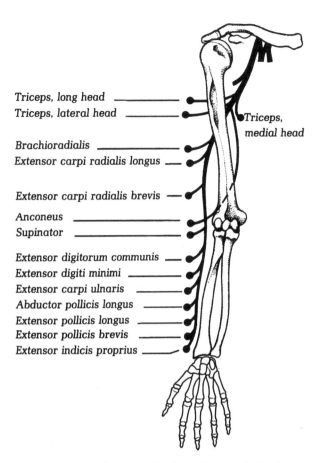

Triceps, long head

Triceps, lateral head

Triceps, medial head

Brachioradialis

Extensor carpi radialis longus

Extensor carpi radialis brevis

Anconeus

Supinator

Extensor digitorum communis

Extensor digiti minimi

Extensor carpi ulnaris

Abductor pollicis longus

Extensor pollicis longus

Extensor pollicis brevis

Extensor indicis proprius

FIG. 3. Radial nerve. Muscles innervated by the radial nerve in the forearm and hand.

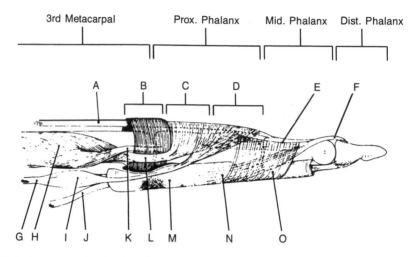

FIG. 4. Anatomy and pathophysiology of the intrinsic muscles and digital extensor mechanism.

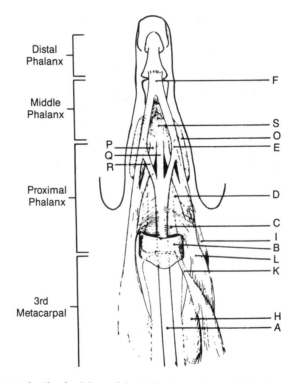

FIG. 5. Anatomy and pathophysiology of the intrinsic muscles and digital extensor mechanism.

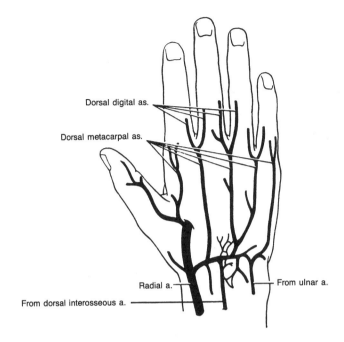

FIG. 6. Dorsal arterial arch.

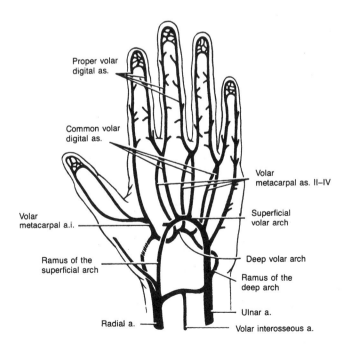

FIG. 7. "Normal" pattern of palmar vascular arches.

Appendix 3

Clinical Assessment Methods

SENSIBILITY

Two-point discrimination, with the use of a blunt instrument, applied in a longitudinal axis of the digit (Fig. 1).

Ratings

1. Normal, less than 6 mm
2. Fair, 6 to 10 mm
3. Poor, 11 to 15 mm
4. Protective, one point perceived
5. Anesthetic, no point perceived

STRENGTH

Grip Strength

Use a squeeze (grip) dynamometer and make three successive determinations. The correct position for recording grip strength is with the arm comfortably at the patient's side, the elbow flexed at 90 degrees, and the forearm and hand resting unsupported. Record and calculate posttreatment percentage relative to pretreatment value as well as to value from the contralateral hand. *Note: This is not a percentage of physical impairment or improvement.*

Pinch Strength

Use a pinch dynamometer. Key pinch is the thumb tip to radial aspect of the middle phalanx of the index finger and is the most universal and preferred value. Record three successive efforts and calculate the average pinch strength

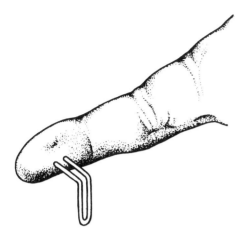

FIG. 1. Two-point discrimination.

or contralateral hand pinch strength. Tip pinch value (reverse key pinch-index tip to ulnar tip of thumb) will be less powerful than key pinch. The recordings are the same as for key pinch. *Note: This is not a percentage of physical impairment.*

MOTION

Total Passive Motion

Sum of angles formed by metacarpophalangeal (MCP), proximal interphalangeal (PIP), and distal interphalangeal (DIP) joints in maximum passive flexion minus the sum of angles of deficit from complete extension at each of these three joints: (MCP + PIP + DIP) – (MCP + PIP + DIP) = total flexion – total extensor lag total passive motion (TPM).

Total Active Motion

Sum of angles formed by MCP, PIP, and DIP joints in maximum active flexion, that is, fist position, minus total extension deficit at the MCP, PIP, and DIP joints with active finger extension (Figs. 2, 3, and 4). Significant hyperextension at any joint, particularly the PIP and DIP joints, is recorded as a deficit in extension and is included in the total extension deficit. Hyperextension must be considered an abnormal value in swan neck (PIP) and boutonniere deformities (DIP). Comparison of pretreatment and posttreatment total active motion (TAM) values will be significant.

Total active motion is a term applied to one finger and is analogous to TPM in calculation except that only active motion is recorded, not passive.

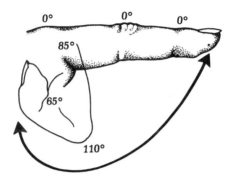

Active	Flexion (°)	Extension (°)
Metacarpophalangeal	85	0
Proximal interphalangeal	110	0
Distal interphalangeal	65	0
Totals	260	0

TAM, Total active motion
260 degrees − 0 degrees = 260 degrees

FIG. 2. Normal.

Stiff MCP +
limited PIP extension

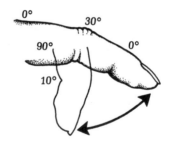

Active	Flexion (°)	Extension (°)
Metacarpophalangeal	0	0
Proximal interphalangeal	90	30
Distal interphalangeal	10	0
Totals	100	30

TAM, Total active motion
100 degrees − 30 degrees = 70 degrees

FIG. 3. Stiff Metacarpophalangeal + Limited Proximal interphalangeal Extension.

Limited MCP + PIP flexion
with good extension

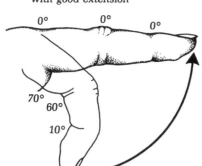

Active	Flexion (°)	Extension Lack (°)
Metacarpophalangeal	70	0
Proximal interphalangeal	60	0
Distal interphalangeal	10	0
Totals	140	0

TAM, Total active motion
140 degrees − 0 degrees = 140 degrees

FIG. 4. Limited MCP + PIP Flexion with Good Extension.

1. Sum of active MCP flexion + active PIP flexion + active DIP flexion.
2. Minus sum of incomplete active extension (if any is present).

It is of critical importance to emphasize that this system of measuring and recording joint motions is used in the following situations:

1. For a single digit
2. To indicate the total motion of that digit in degrees
3. To compare this to subsequent measurements of that same digit or the corresponding normal digit of the opposite hand in the same patient to determine if the patient is gaining or losing motion

It is not intended for the following:

1. To calculate a percentage of "functional improvement or loss"
2. To calculate a "percentage of impairment"

VASCULAR STATUS

Patients who have vascular repair are evaluated in the following manner.

Subjective

1. Assessment of "coldness"

Objective

1. Capillary refill; normal ≤ 2 seconds
2. Turgor or fullness of the tip
3. Venous congestion
4. Allen's test
5. Digital Allen's test

Other Noninvasive Methods of Assessment

1. Doppler examination of the hand
   —General exam
   —Doppler test
   —Allen's test
2. Skin temperature
3. Pulse oximetry

Other Methods of Assessment

1. Magnetic resonance angiography
2. Transfemoral arteriography

Subject Index

Page numbers followed by f refer to figures; page numbers followed by t refer to tables.